# Avoiding Burnout Working Women

Vital Warnings to Extinguish Burnout Before It Even Happens

Ruth D.D.R.

© Copyright 2022 - All rights reserved.

The content contained within this book may not be reproduced, duplicated or transmitted without direct written permission from the author or the publisher.

Under no circumstances will any blame or legal responsibility be held against the publisher, or author, for any damages, reparation, or monetary loss due to the information contained within this book, either directly or indirectly.

## Legal Notice:

This book is copyright protected. It is only for personal use. You cannot amend, distribute, sell, use, quote or paraphrase any part, or the content within this book, without the consent of the author or publisher.

## Disclaimer Notice:

Please note the information contained within this document is for educational and entertainment purposes only. All effort has been executed to present accurate, up to date, reliable, complete information. No warranties of any kind are declared or implied. Readers acknowledge that the author is not engaged in the rendering of legal, financial, medical or professional advice. The content within this book has been derived from various sources. Please consult a licensed professional before attempting any techniques outlined in this book.

By reading this document, the reader agrees that under no circumstances is the author responsible for any losses, direct or indirect, that are incurred as a result of the use of the information contained within this document, including, but not limited to, errors, omissions, or inaccuracies.

# Table of Contents

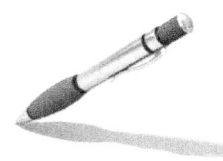

Chapter 1 Life Is a Cycle; So Is Stress .................................................. 1

Chapter 2 Is It Stress or Am I Burning Out? ............................... 19

Chapter 3 Getting to Know Your Body and Mind ................ 37

Chapter 4 Finding Your Coping Mechanism ....................... 54

Chapter 5 Time Management Made Easy ................................ 72

Chapter 6 Mindfulness—Blocking Out Burnout Once and for All ............................................................................................. 92

Chapter 7 Enjoy Your Job Again ..................................................... 105

Conclusion ............................................................................................. 119

Accepting Yourself .............................................................................. 121

References .............................................................................................. 124

# Introduction

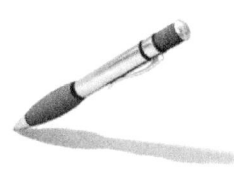

You know those moments where you have a never-ending to-do list, and no matter how hard you try, you just can't seem to get anything done? This is usually met with the feelings of high stress and anxiety, that growing feeling deep within your rib cage that feels like your heart is fluttering, and the heat is swelling to the back of your throat. You keep ignoring it and pushing it back down and keep trying to rise back up at any opportunity. You're absolutely exhausted; you're frustrated; and you're trying your hardest to be a good mom, a good partner, a good employee or worker, and just an all-round good human being, but no matter how much you try, you find things are moving too fast. You can't keep up. And then, before you know it, you finally *snap*!

This is a feeling I am all too familiar with, not just having experienced it myself, but I have seen so many other women experience it too. They have often also tried to put into words what they were feeling, but it was to no avail. It is, after all, a difficult feeling to describe unless you know the feeling yourself. How do you describe the physical, emotional, and mental experiences of stress? Whether these women have thought that no one would understand or they were afraid to admit this feeling, I have watched these feelings drop even the strongest woman to her knees in crippling stress, anxiety, and exhaustion.

The scary thing about experiencing these emotions is that it seems almost sudden. One second, I am on top of everything: Everything at home is running like a well-oiled machine, the house is tidy, and everything is perfectly organized. I am on top of every school event: attending every hockey game or soccer match and attending every PTA meeting with freshly baked cupcakes; I have attended and prepared every meeting at the office and still made it home on time to cook a wholesome family dinner. And then the next second, my plate is too full, I feel like I am drowning, and I can't keep track of anything. It is as if, in an instant, things changed. But how? I just had everything under control. No. When I looked back, that was actually three weeks ago, and in the midst of the chaos, everything seemed to fly by. I had taken on too much and under the weight of my own high expectations. I had fallen.

All of a sudden, I can't get out of bed, I constantly feel touched out by my kids, and showering seems like a task I just can't seem to bring myself to do. Unfortunately, it wasn't until I was in the thick of it, experiencing these intense emotions at excessively high levels, that I realized what this strange sensation was—burnout. Burnout is a strange thing; it can make you feel weak and isolated because you do so much; and no one ever gives you the slightest nod of acknowledgment for what you have done, even when, sometimes, that is all you need. You always do the job perfectly that you have set the bar of expectation extremely high for yourself. People never wonder what goes into the work that you do; they just know it's going to be perfect all the time. Talk about high pressure, right? You feel like the 24 hours that each new day brings just never is enough. And once you finally finish the task that's at hand, there are going to be 20 new ones waiting for you.

Well, I'm here to help you nip those feelings in the bud, because you don't know you're experiencing burnout until you're completely and entirely burnt out and scrambling to find a way of bouncing back.

No, you are not irrationally emotional; you're not just going through the motions and stressors of everyday life; it most definitely is not normal; and you are not the only one! Sometimes, hearing that you are not alone and that you are not the only one who has experienced this is all the comfort you need. It gives you the confidence and power of thinking, *If they can do it, then so can I!*

Shall I let you in on a secret? Burnout is not a picky eater. It can affect anyone if you allow yourself to take on more than you can handle. The mom who seems to have it all together at your child's school, who juggles work and home life seamlessly, and who seems to have the most helpful partner in the world, may have experienced burnout before. The corporate businesswoman who seems to run the company better than the owners of the company, she too has probably experienced burnout. The work-from-home mom who always seems to have time to play with her kids, she has also experienced burnout. Burnout does not discriminate, and it doesn't pick and choose who its next target will be.

While it is all well and good to read a simple blog post on the experiences associated with burnout and how to know the signs of burnout, the advice isn't exactly the same as hearing it from the horse's mouth, so to say. This may have been a great tool in helping you figure out the road you're heading down and helped you figure out that you may be getting burnt out, and that has ultimately led you here.

Through this book, I aim to achieve three goals. The first goal I hope to achieve is to destigmatize the idea of being burnt out. I hope to change the narrative that you and others may have toward being burnt out. I hope to prove to you that being burnt out does not mean you're a failure, that it's okay to not be the superwoman that society somehow expects all women to so effortless embody, and that being burnt out, or reaching that point, doesn't mean you're weak, and it most certainly does not mean you're a hard worker.

Next, I hope to equip you with the tools you need to know what the early signs of burnout are so that you may use the strategies I present in this book to mitigate it before it even happens. If you've had chicken pox, you aren't likely to ever contract it again from someone who has it. Unfortunately, burnout is not a one-off deal like chicken pox. You can get burnt out multiple times. So even if you have experienced it before, I am here to help guide you and help you avoid experiencing it again.

Next, this book aims to guide you and provide strategies to not only avoid burnout but how to overcome burnout once you're in it. As I said before, before you know it, you're out of your depths, and you're right in the center of this horrible and overwhelming experience. While it is great to equip yourself with the tools to avoid experiencing burnout, perhaps you, or someone else, need a hand to be pulled out of the depths of the bottomless pit of burnout.

Lastly, through the strategies that I have employed myself, I hope to share with you mechanisms that will help you find yourself, learn to say no when things are too much to bear, and show you that self-love is a necessity, not a luxury. As every woman needs to learn the fine line that balances work life and home life, this book will help guide you in ways that balances all facets of your life that are perfect for you.

# Chapter 1

# Life Is a Cycle; So Is Stress

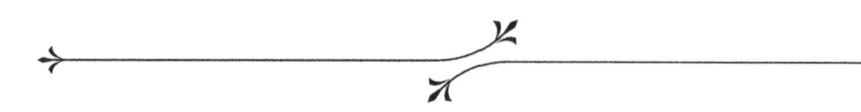

One of the most frustrating things I have ever heard is, "Just stop stressing," or "Don't stress about it." I keep thinking that if it were that simple, no one would ever experience stress. No one goes about their day hoping they experience some sort of negative feeling—which is what stress is. But stress is an uncontrollable hormonal response created by our body.

With stress being a hormonal response, it is an innate chemical reaction to our surroundings. We can't control it anymore than we can control our shivering, which is also a response to a cold environment. The only way we can stop ourselves from stressing is by removing ourselves from a stressful environment. But a lot of the time, as with work, we have difficulty in separating our work lives from our home lives, and our stresses from the day seem to follow us back home.

Now, imagine this scenario: It has been an exceptionally long day at the office, there was a misunderstanding, and something went wrong, leaving you scrambling to pick up the pieces and solve a major problem. There were back-to-back meetings, some related to the catastrophe you were trying to resolve and others that were scheduled. On your way home, you were stuck in excessive traffic which led to even further frustrations, and then you got home and realized that you didn't take any chicken out of the freezer to defrost. This seemingly small thing sent you over the edge. But why? Because as with everyone else in the world, you couldn't magically leave the stress of the day at the door before you entered your home.

But as with anything in this wonderful and natural world, in order to mitigate something and gain better control of it, we need to better understand how it works and why.

Let's start at the beginning. What is stress? Stress is a physical or an emotional response to a stressor. Stress in itself is not an emotion, but it can cause you to experience an array of specific emotions such as frustration, anger, and even fear. There are two main types of stress. The first is acute stress which is the type that lasts for a very short while, such as when you are about to go for a ride on a roller coaster or you almost slip and fall. It is the type of stress that accompanies excitement and is our body's way of keeping ourselves out of harm's way. Acute stress is also a healthy form of stress, and no one is excluded from feeling it. The second type of stress is chronic stress, and this is the one that is not good for you. This is the type of stress that goes on for a long period of time (MedlinePlus, 2020).

As an example, I once experienced chronic stress when I worked at my last place of employment. My direct superior was someone who purposefully made my life hard. I loved my work, but I hated my job. I dreaded waking up in the morning, but I stuck with it. That is, until I started experiencing health problems, excessive headaches, hair loss, and extreme fatigue because of the persistent stress I was experiencing. Chronic stress, if not handled correctly, can pose serious mental and physical health problems.

Sometimes, our chronic stress is so consistent in our lives that we get used to it. When it is so consistent and persistent, we are in a constant state of stress, and we don't get to complete our stress cycles. Yes, you read that correctly. Stress happens in cycles known as stress reaction cycles. Contrary to what we have been led to believe in the past, stress happens in a cycle where you start at one point and make your way through the entire process and ultimately recover from it. But if you are constantly facing stress, it makes completing a cycle nearly impossible, and that is when stress becomes unhealthy (*Stress Cycles,* 2020).

This means that there is no one way to fix or remedy the stress that you are facing, but rather, there are multiple opportunities to interrupt the stress cycle at any point before it becomes entirely debilitating and begins having detrimental effects on you. These are the different stages within a stress cycle:

1. The external stressor. A buzzword that I am sure you have heard many times before is "trigger." It is something that sets off a response, not always positive, in your mind that results in stress. And the thing that triggers you is known as a stressor. This can be anything from someone cutting you off in traffic to your child throwing a tantrum in the middle of a shopping center. It is here in the stress cycle where the external element is solely at play and you are merely the experiencer. However, as the experiencer, you develop ways to deal with, cope with, and respond to this external stressor (Samartano, 2018).

2. The internal appraisal. Once you have experienced the external stimulus from a stressor or a triggering event, your mind and body then need to take a tally of what is happening and how it plans to respond to what is happening. This can happen usually before, during, or immediately after the external stressor has been experienced. As with all other animals and mammals, our body is designed for survival. Even though we do not live in the wild, our senses are useful in making sure we are aware of our surroundings and that we keep ourselves safe. But even beyond our senses, our instinct plays a big role in keeping us safe. This instinct and sense are prompted firstly by our amygdala, which receives the perceived danger from our senses. The amygdala controls emotions such as fear and pleasure, and once this is activated, it activates the hypothalamus and the pituitary gland which is responsible for maintaining homeostasis, or internal balance, in our body. The hypothalamus and the pituitary gland pass messages on to the rest of the body through the autonomic nervous system which controls our breathing, heart rate, and blood pressure (Samartano, 2018).

3. Physiological responses. By this point, all of the reactions you are having to stress are happening almost behind the scenes where you are not consciously aware of it. It is all occurring internally. Once the hypothalamus and the pituitary gland sense that this is an external stimulus presenting danger, it activates the sympathetic nervous system, which is what governs the fight-or-flight impulse. Next, your adrenal glands are activated, and they get ready to respond by preparing to release adrenaline and cortisol. The fight-or-flight response stimulates the cardiovascular system and the musculoskeletal system which increases your heart rate, sending more blood to your extremities and allowing your body to decide if it is going to fight or flee. It is important to note that when your sympathetic nervous system is activated, your parasympathetic nervous system is disabled. The parasympathetic nervous system essentially controls digestion and rest. You are then left in a state of hyperarousal (Samartano, 2018).
4. Internalization. This is the point in the stress cycle where you actively begin to realize that you are experiencing stress. It may not always be obvious, but you may begin experiencing feelings of anxiety,

fear, and dread. In more immediate danger, you may find your heart pounding in your chest and your palms being extremely sweaty.
5. Maladaptive coping. As the stress becomes more apparent and you begin experiencing its physical and emotional manifestations, you begin looking for ways to cope with this stress. Depending on how excessive the stress may be and if it is ongoing, the methods you may choose to ease your stress can either ease your stress or make it far worse. In times of excessive stress and distress, people may turn to drugs, alcohol, excessive scrolling through social media, or food, or it can be behavioral where you find yourself extremely hyperactive or fatigued and even throwing yourself deeper into work. Maladaptive coping mechanisms are not the best approach to mitigating and alleviating stress.

Looking at the stress cycle as mentioned above, it is easy to see that stress does not start and end at the exact moment you start seeing the physical effects of it. It is an entire cycle, and depending on the type of stressor or stimulus that you receive, it can either last for a long time, or it can last for a short period of time.

For example, if you are walking down the road and a car almost bumps you, you will go through the entire stress cycle as mentioned above, but it will be a lot quicker. You will be shocked and probably shaking for a few hours, but once your hormone levels drop back to normal, you will find yourself calm once again, and slowly, the event will fade, not from your memory but from constantly replaying in your head. It will not fade from your memory because your mind will make sure you don't allow yourself to get into that position again. You may find yourself consciously walking far from the actual street next time because you remember the time a car almost bumped you, or you may find yourself looking left and right many more times before actually crossing. Once again, the brain has provided you with a new survival tactic related specifically to an incident that had previously occurred.

However, in contrast to this, if you find yourself experiencing prolonged stress, you may be in a downward spiral toward burnout without even knowing it. For example, if you are placed in a situation where you have a bad relationship with a family member and you need to see them often, you may find yourself dreading the weekends or whenever it is that you usually see them. Seeing them, or even knowing that you are going to see them, is the trigger that you experience. If you see this person often enough, you may not have fully recovered from your previous stress cycle before the next one begins.

While the trigger remains the same, your body is in a physiologically heightened phase consistently. If you don't overcome the third phase of the stress cycle which is the physiological response, your body remains in a state of hyperarousal for long periods of time. You live in a state of fight or flight, and your parasympathetic nervous system is inhibited for long periods of time, making digestion and rest harder to attain. Basically, if your stress cycle remains constant at the third stage of the cycle, your body will begin harming itself because of the physical environment you find yourself in.

Additionally, if your stress cycle remains incomplete at stage four, you may find yourself in a constant state of internal and mental negativity. You may begin questioning your abilities, feeling like a failure, and dreading doing a task or an activity, which may result in you feeling like an overall bad person. Going back to the example of seeing family members that are a trigger for your stress, you may find yourself trying to convince yourself that you are seeing them every week for your children to be with your family. If you try to avoid the situation, you may find yourself feeling like a bad parent or a selfish parent. We often underestimate the power of our internal voice. It is the voice we live with day in and day out. If that internal voice is telling us negative things, it won't be long before we start believing it. If the greatest influence in your life, which is yourself, is telling you that you are not good at something or that you can't do something, chances are that you will begin living up—or living down—to the standard you have of yourself.

And this inevitably leads to the fifth stage of the cycle—developing maladaptive coping mechanisms. Maladaptive coping mechanisms are those that we form to help us fit better into a specific environment. It could be needing to drink excessive amounts of coffee before leaving to a job that causes you stress, it could be smoking as a way to relieve the consistent stress you feel, or it could even be needing excessive amounts of alcohol before you leave to an event because you need to get to a point where you can bear being in such an environment without succumbing to your stress. If you develop a negative maladaptive coping mechanism, you could find yourself becoming dependent on this negative mechanism. Smoking, alcohol, and any form of drugs, whether it is medical or nonmedical, can all have detrimental effects on your health, especially if you are using it to numb some sort of ongoing stress. But you could also develop certain behavioral aspects that are detrimental to your well-being. You may find yourself thrown into work, overeating, and not exercising, all of which can burn you out.

Knowing where you are within the stress cycle may help you develop techniques to overcome the stress that you are feeling. It will help in disrupting prolonged experiences of the stress cycle, and it will lead to you finding better coping mechanisms, rather than those mechanisms that will negatively impact you.

## **Stress and Stressors**

Whether you are experiencing extreme stress from your everyday activities such as being a mother or from your job or whether you have just experienced an immediate effect of stress, there always seems to be something that can cause us stress. Generally, stress may be caused by anything that we perceive as new, as a complete surprise that has caught us off guard, when we feel threatened, or even when we have little control over a situation (Mental Health Foundation, 2021). As humans, we tend to have a need to control what is happening around us. That is why we are also creatures of habit and routine. When we know what to expect, we can prepare for it, and this makes us more confident in our routine and the duties we are hoping to complete. Even from very young ages, children prefer to know a routine. They may even become grumpy and frustrated if they are taken out of their routine. I have noticed, when my children were very young, that after a week of strict routine where each day looked quite similar to the previous day in terms of structure, when the weekend rolled in, my kids were fussy and all around more grumpy than usual. Monday to Friday, they went to school, nap time was the same, and while they may have been doing different activities each day, the general structure and time that they did certain activities remained the same. On a weekend, we are always out and about, running errands and doing things that took them out of their routine. They often missed nap times and acted out because of it. But this was no fault of theirs. I too found myself getting frustrated when my routine was interrupted well into adulthood. As an example, during one of my work days, our entire neighborhood experienced a power outage. I lost half the day of work as I couldn't get anything done without electricity. This left me feeling entirely overwhelmed and stressed out, and my whole routine was set off track.

But even with all the negativity and being surrounded by stress, it does have some positive aspects. Have you noticed how you're somehow able to push out almost double or triple the amount of work that you would on an ordinary day when you have a deadline looming? Have you noticed how you manage to take on super speed and precision when you're walking alone in a parking lot? Have you ever wondered where you learned certain driving skills that have saved you from a car accident? All of these incidents were the result of stress that helped us in achieving precision and safety. Because, essentially, our goal as human beings is to maintain our survival. Stress also helps us to adjust rapidly when we do face unexpected changes. For example, if we look back in the instance where I was unable to work due to a power outage, I had to come up with a way to adapt so I didn't lose out on the time I had. I couldn't cook because the power was out, but I knew I needed to run errands the next day. What I did instead was I headed out to run those errands and I ordered take out for my family as well, and I tried to make up for lost time the next day. While it wasn't the ideal situation and it, by no means, adhered to the plan I had for that particular day, I still managed to adapt.

Through the internal release of cortisol, our body triggers off a way for us to survive. But what happens if your body experiences too much cortisol? With cortisol being the primary stress hormone in your body, it can lead to a number of physical and mental deficits if you release too much. First, looking at the physical, cortisol can have a number of impacts on your physical health if you produce too much or too little. Producing too little cortisol, or having too little present in your body, could lead to changes and discoloration in your skin, weight loss, loss of appetite, and low blood pressure. Unfortunately, having too little cortisol isn't as easy to fix as giving yourself a good old fright. You may need to get medical treatment in the form of dexamethasone, hydrocortisone, or prednisone (Cassoobhoy, 2017).

However, if you are constantly under stress and experience high levels of cortisol, you may experience symptoms that lead to Cushing's syndrome which leads to weight gain, bruises easily appearing on the skin, diabetes, and overall muscle weakness (Cassoobhoy,

2017). In addition, you may find yourself experiencing cardiovascular symptoms, digestive issues, and an overall weaker immune system. Experiencing too much cortisol can even affect your relationships and your overall functioning.

In relationships, it has been found that, in high-stress situations, couples tend to fight over things that would normally be resolved quite peacefully. This is because stress triggers emotions such as anger, irritation, and frustration (Lawson, n.d.). Do you know the feeling of coming home from a long day at the office and having to pick up the kids, prepare dinner, put them in the bath, and get them ready for bed? At this point, you are tired and exhausted, and stress about tomorrow has already started to seep in. And almost anything your partner does, or does not do, can set you off. If the stress is excessive, you may begin experiencing feelings of resentment toward your partner if they are just sitting around and doing nothing. You may feel that you are taking on the entire load of your work stresses and your home stresses, and while this may be valid, you may find your children just being needy for you and not wanting your partner to do anything for them. But this doesn't take your feelings away. It could even be that your partner asks you for a cup of coffee in the midst of your mind being a twirling whirlwind, and that can lead to an outburst that may later even be dubbed as an overreaction.

At that moment, it is hard to find rationality beyond your actions. All you know is that you are frustrated and you don't know why. This puts a strain on a relationship by creating an argument and adding further stress on you when it could have been entirely avoided.

Stress impacting your job is another strange occurrence. The thing that is strange about this is that, a lot of the time, it is our jobs that cause us stress, but when we become extremely stressed out, we find it difficult to do our job. This turns into a monstrous cycle of us being stressed by our job and being inefficient in our job, which makes us more stressed. You know the feeling of having a deadline around the corner? This is enough to cause you stress because you have found yourself procrastinating, uncertain, or even nervous. This leads to you experiencing debilitating stress. Perhaps you are now unable to work because you have an aching tummy or a headache. Perhaps you dread waking up in the morning and having to go to work. Maybe you even try calling in sick or have outbursts in the office. All of these are the things that further makes you inefficient at work and leads to further stress (Lawson, n.d.).

All of these things that make your heart pound and make your breathing fast are all considered stressors. The thing about stressors, however, is that it is different for everyone, meaning there is no one-size-fits-all remedy for stressors. Yes, you can remedy the stress that you feel and implement strategies to reduce the stress, but the thing that causes the stress will still be there. Anything that could be perceived as a danger is considered a stressor. If we look at different scenarios, we can better understand what a stressor is to different people. First, we can look at someone who gets extremely stressed out by cooking. I know this may seem like a silly thing to get stressed about, but for some, cooking is not just something that brings them joy but is actually a very strenuous task. For this person, heading to a restaurant where they experience an immersive experience watching others cook over an open flame may even be a stressor. For children, loud noises may scare them because they perceive it as a danger. If you shout at a child or if you take them to an arcade where there are excessively loud noises, the child may suffer from sensory overload and experience heightened stress. Once again, going back to the stressful experience of visiting family members, perhaps there is one person that stresses you out the most. Whether it is because of the excessive negativity that a person emits or because of past trauma that you are trying to overcome, that person is a stressor to you.

While some people use the words "stress" and "stressor" interchangeably, they are not the same thing. One is the cause, and the other is a reaction. A stressor can be psychological—this is a stress that takes place in your mind such as a deadline that is around the corner or your oven burning out just before you host

Thanksgiving dinner. The other stress is physical—this is what happens if you experience a traumatic injury after a car accident or the stress your body goes through physically when you fight off a cold or flu.

There are many ways that you can relieve stress, from getting out into nature, meditating, eating healthier, and getting some exercise to speaking to others, taking a break from a stressful daily routine, and seeing a therapist. But while these are all tactics that you can use to treat stress once you are already in the stress cycle, it is not a way of reducing a stressor. Essentially, a stressor is not something that can be remedied or reduced because it is anything that we perceive as a danger. But do not fret. All is not lost. There are effective ways not only to avoid your stressors but also to find strategies to better adapt and reduce the perceived danger from certain stressors.

The first thing you need to do is find out what is a stressor for you. Once you have identified and pinpointed what it is, you can start devising strategies that help ease the stress. The stressor is not your office building or doing your job as an accountant, but rather, your stressor may be the mountain of paperwork and administration that comes along with being an accountant. Perhaps carrying out phone calls to clients may be your stressor. Once you have identified it, you can try to mitigate the problem. Trust me, avoidance is not the solution. If your stressor is the mountain of paperwork that takes you away from working with numbers, which is what you love doing, then perhaps you can devise an administrative timetable which allows you to chip away at managing daily administrative tasks for short periods of time, rather than leaving it to build up and catch up with you at the end of the day. If conducting phone calls is your stressor, then you may implement a strategy where you work collaboratively with a receptionist or with someone who doesn't have a problem carrying out phone calls, and they can assist you in the stressful task.

However, it is important to note that, just in the same way as you can't avoid a stressor entirely, you can't pass the duty or responsibility to others. If it is something that you can avoid, such as a particular road or intersection that causes you way too much stress and anxiety when driving, you could leave a bit earlier to avoid that stressor and take another route. In this case, avoidance may help. But if it is part of your job responsibility, you need to find appropriate coping mechanisms, such as time management, counseling, and seeking assistance from others.

## Chapter 2

# Is It Stress or Am I Burning Out?

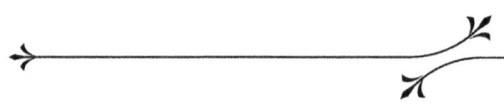

"I'm burnt out."

"This is burning me out. I just can't cope anymore."

**Burnout**. This is the word that we have heard many times before. Often, it gets thrown around without truly understanding the meaning or the feelings associated with this term. I can guarantee and assure you now that it has nothing to do with a fever, illness, or even your oven.

So what exactly is burnout? The concept has probably existed since the dawn of time, for as long as humans would have had to work and for as long as their work has been a cause of stress. However, despite it existing for a long time, it has only recently become something noteworthy or has become something that is worth a name. In 1975, German psychologist Herbert Freudenberger developed the term "burnout" which he used to refer to certain symptoms he was noticing in professionals, mostly at clinics or alternative self-help institutes (Freudenberger, 1975). The prominent symptoms that he noticed were feelings of failure and exhaustion owing to high demands on the individual from their place of work. However, since Freudenberger formally established the concept of burnout, there have been many other theories that have been brought about which ineffectually describe the concept. Most of these theories or definitions have been based around the causes, the results, or the physiological, behavioral, and physical manifestation of burnout, rather than the actual definition of it.

According to the World Health Organization (WHO, 2019), burnout is not a medical condition but is rather "a syndrome conceptualized as resulting from chronic workplace stress that has not been successfully managed." The WHO (2019) further states that burnout is specifically related to the occupational area of our lives and can not be applied to any other context. This means that you can't be burnt out from anything other than work. But because the term has gained so much traction in recent years, we may find people using the term freely to apply to different aspects of their lives. Some may say that their daily commute is burning them out. While their daily commute may make them feel stressed, frustrated, or exhausted, by definition, it cannot burn them out. However, this doesn't mean that burnout only affects the professional sphere of your life. No, burnout seeps and bleeds into every facet of your life that causes you to feel excessively overwhelmed. Perhaps you're burnt out from work, and the commute is a stressor or a trigger that you try to avoid.

The WHO further classifies burnout by three specific components:

1) Someone who suffers from burnout will experience physical manifestations in the form of fatigue, having little to no energy, and absolute exhaustion. As with many struggles that people face mentally, it does begin to show physically, and the same is true for burnout. Just because it is not something tangible, doesn't mean it won't affect you physically. Experiencing extreme sensations of tiredness can make you feel demotivated and impact your overall outlook and approach to certain aspects of your life. This can result in a notable change in your performance as burnout increases and your mental health declines.

2) You may find yourself experiencing intense cynicism toward your job, heightened feelings of negativity, and feeling mentally removed from your job. This could be the mind's defense mechanism against things we have a negative feeling toward—you try to neglect that thing and do whatever you can to gain some distance. This is something that I, too, have experienced. It was at a time when I was burnt out but I didn't even know it. I was overworked, underpaid, and ready to move on to new ventures. I decided to take the leap and hand in my resignation. While working through my notice period, and even before that, perhaps from the moment I made the decision to leave, I had absolutely no interest in the job. I dreaded and loathed every email ping and every phone call that came to me during that notice period. I was distant, not just from my job but from every aspect of it. I had even distanced myself from my colleagues because of the negativity that I was experiencing. It wasn't that the people around me were negative or giving off a negative energy, but rather, it was just my feelings toward the job that I was hoping to depart from.
3) You will likely experience a reduced professional efficacy level. I'm sure you know the feeling of having something that you just don't feel like doing. When I think of something that I really don't want to do, it is usually washing, drying, and packing the dishes or folding and packing laundry. These are tasks that,

even if I was sitting around and doing absolutely nothing, I still wouldn't want to tackle. But when these feelings are associated with your job and take place in the professional sphere, you may find yourself slowly slipping down the success ladder. But why are you less productive when you're burnt out? Well, remember the fight-or-flight hormone that we previously mentioned? When your body experiences a constant influx of this stress hormone, it may feel like it's constantly running at full steam ahead. These invisible processes that are running in the background are a lot for your body to handle, and that is why after a stressful day or event, you find yourself feeling exhausted. Now, if this stress is not limited to one day but goes on for weeks and weeks, you could only imagine that every day is spent fighting a seemingly losing battle to exhaustion and decreased productivity. But this reduction in your professional efficacy doesn't just affect you. It is through this that you see the effects of burnout trickling all through an organization if one person suffers. Reduced productivity will affect the entire organization as well, and you may find deadlines missed, you may find clients experiencing dissatisfaction with a service, and you may experience an overall decline in output, which leads to a decline in profitability.

While burnout may have been incorrectly labeled in the past, the description of causes and manifestations of burnout have provided experts with a great way of breaking down the associated concepts and equipping people with ways to protect themselves against burnout. Looking first at the causes of burnout, there was a clear need to fill a void of the occurrence of extreme stress associated with work. In all facets of life, we experience varying forms of stress. A great source of stress is parenting. You constantly question if you are doing a good job, every tantrum or outburst makes you wonder if you are ruining your child, and just when you think you have a hang of it—your child is eating well and doing well at school—they get sick, and your stress skyrockets once again. We also experience financial stress, the stress of just not knowing how you're going to make it to your next payday. And this often leads to other forms of stress and pressure in that it may affect your relationships, your family dynamic, and cause arguments in your home. So with all these existing forms of stress that exist in the world and with the prominence of professional stress that the world has seen, work stress needed its own name.

## Causes of Burnout

The causes of burnout have been conceptualized, and while they are flexible in that different people may experience different causes, these have been found to be the most notable and the most common causes. One of the most prominent and notable causes is having little to no control. This means that you have no say or influence in your own job. If you think of the normal nine-to-five corporate office job where people are micromanaged by a large variety of managerial titles, chances are your job is laid out for you, your schedule is laid out for you, your deadlines have been laid out for you, and no consideration is made for individual variance. This means that everyone is given the same workload, despite each person's strengths and weaknesses. However, the work dynamic in recent years has seen a phenomenal change. With the onset of the COVID-19 pandemic, companies had to relinquish control and develop some sort of trust with their employees. Employees started working from home, and they received more control, but "traditional" measures of management were no longer successful despite management trying to hold the reins. As things have been gradually starting to go back to normal and with traditional, work-from-home, or hybrid methods of operations being implemented, employees realized the causes of their burnout, and they realized that they would rather control their own lives. Companies that refused to adapt began facing something we now call the Great Resignation, which started in the beginning of 2021, whereby employees voluntarily left their jobs. People quickly realized the benefits of freelancing or being your own boss and the benefits that it had on their mental health as well.

Another cause of burnout is a lack of social support. This is something that seeps deeper into your personal life. The feeling of isolation is extremely overwhelming. If you feel like you don't have support in your workplace or at home, chances are you will feel alone. These feelings of isolation could stem from feeling like you don't have any support in your workplace. If you face challenges at work and you don't have anyone that you can turn to for assistance, if your requests for assistance are met with negative feelings, or even if you feel like you need to be worried about your job at every turn, you may be lacking social support in your workplace. But this lack of support can even come from spaces outside of your work. Maybe among your friends, you feel as though, in comparison, you are a lot less successful than your friends or if you feel that they don't support your job. I have seen a lot of career women crumble at the hands of their partner, with unrealistic expectations placed on them which made them feel unsupported in their jobs. As a woman, so much responsibility falls into your hands. You are required to be an outstanding employee and an outstanding mother and wife. Once again, traditionalism requires a woman to come home and cook and take care of her kids, despite being at work all day. Partners who conform to these traditionalist worldviews may find themselves arguing with the women in their lives when they feel that work is taking priority.

Another noteworthy cause of burnout is a lack of work–life balance. Work–life balance is something I have heard thrown about a lot. People are implored to strike this ideal balance, and they are told that, when the clock hits 5:00 p.m., you need to clock out and power down to focus on your family and your personal life. As great and as wonderful as this sounds, not many people have the ability, or the capacity, to strike this balance. If someone works a job that is very deadline-specific, they may find themselves working overtime. This can quickly develop into a habit whereby people work overtime and have little or no time to spend at home with their families. Also, just because you have physically clocked out from work, does not mean you can immediately switch your mind off and stop thinking about work. Lastly, while a lot of people may try to maintain some sort of work–life balance, other people may not respect those boundaries. This may lead to people calling after hours and discussing work during evening phone calls which is never beneficial.

We are always encouraged to maintain a long tenure at certain jobs or places of employment. It is said that this forms a wonderful reputation and surrounds you with an air of loyalty and commitment when you do decide to move on to another job. However, when you are faced with spending years in a job that is completely monotonous or extremely chaotic, you may find this to be another cause of burnout. In a chaotic job and in an extremely quiet or boring job, the amount of energy you need to maintain a specific level of focus is extremely high. This high demand for focus can lead to mental fatigue and, if done so for prolonged periods of time, can lead to burnout. A lot of movies have shown us great depictions of these two extremities of chaos and monotony. We have seen librarian jobs as quiet, still, and having the same morose feeling surrounding daily operations consistently, then we have seen the wild and loud, adrenaline-fueled operations of the stock markets. These portrayals in film, although dramatized, show us the overwhelming state of these two extremities. And just by watching a few minutes of these operations on the big screen is enough to induce anxiety.

## Emotional, Physical, and Mental Signs of Burnout

The concept of burnout is quite an extraordinary one. It shows us the intricacies of our body and of our fundamental makeup as a human. It shows us how the internal can be so powerful that it runs over and manifests in the physical. Although burnout happens internally, it is not something we know we are experiencing until the physical manifestations begin to appear. So how do you know what to look for and to know you are experiencing burnout? People are so different, and two people may experience burnout in very different ways. First, let us look at the emotional signs of burnout.

We all aspire to exude confidence in our endeavors, whether we actually are confident or whether we fake it until we make it (which often leads to intense feelings of imposter syndrome). Either way, confidence plays a big role in all of our endeavors. Confidence is an emotion, a feeling of being able to achieve or accomplish what you set your mind to or that the path you have chosen will lead to a desired state. When you are on the road to experiencing burnout, as your stress increases, you may find yourself feeling less and less confident toward your ability to carry out your job successfully. You may have started out doing really well and experienced positive feedback from those around you. But if you make a mistake or a slipup because you are overworked and extremely stressed, your confidence level can rapidly decrease.

As all of the elements of stress culminate and come to a head and you begin feeling overwhelmed about your capabilities at work, you may find yourself feeling disconnected from a job you once liked. I once had a friend that worked in a corporate job. She enjoyed her job but was at a dead end with no financial growth prospects at the company she was employed at. So she decided to expand her horizons and move on to something better. She found another job fairly quickly given her experience and expertise, and it provided her with the financial stability she was hoping for. But after three weeks in the new job, she had grown to despise it. The workload was far higher, her boss would sit on her neck requiring hourly updates of her progress, she had no time to think or breathe, and she often came home with work to finish, resulting in her losing valuable time with her children and her husband. She had grown to loathe her job, she didn't even look forward to waking up in the morning, and even the successful completion of a project with great feedback from her clients meant absolutely nothing to her. That major disconnect from her job, where positive or negative feedback meant nothing, is a point that many experience when they are on the verge of or fully experiencing burnout—but they don't know it.

With all these emotions that begin clouding and shrouding your mind, you may end up having an all-around negative approach to your job and even to your career. Now, there needs to be a distinct line drawn between what your job is and what your career is. A job is what you do for money, but a career is what you focus your mind and your desires on, it is what you consistently work toward and what you set goals toward achieving. I have a friend who had placed this in a very nice context. She said that her job is working as a barista. She needs money to study and to ultimately build her career, which is to be a writer. She was working toward a degree in literature at the time of working as a barista, because writing and words were her passion. Writing was a career that she was striving toward; she had goals set in place about where she wanted to be in her writing career in two, five, and ten years down the line. It was her passion. She then went on to say that the moment your job and your career intersect is the moment that you truly begin to enjoy the professional aspect of your life. This, according to her, is where job satisfaction truly lies.

However, if your job is getting in the way of your career, you may experience burnout before you even have the chance to work on your goals and on achieving your career. Burnout can ultimately stand in the way of your motivation of working toward your career; it can stand in the way of you even trying to move on from the job that is weighing you down. And if you have no one to speak to, which it may often seem like, you may begin to feel lonely in your struggles. I have often seen people try to avoid sharing the stresses and dissatisfaction they have in their jobs because they have so often been met with the response of, "Well, you should be glad you have a job at all, because in this economic climate, not many people are as lucky as you are." Yes, this is true. Financially, the world is in a tough place, but when it comes to affecting your mental health and sharing how you feel toward your job, no one should be shut down. Loneliness, and feeling like you're going through something by yourself, can be the hardest feeling anyone may face.

All of the abovementioned emotional signs of burnout ultimately leaves people feeling one thing—the urge of wanting to give up. We have all felt this at some point or the other. You feel like curling up on the bed and drifting into a deep sleep, hoping that for the next few days, no one will need you or want you. You find yourself hoping to take some days away from work, from being a mom, from doing the things you are normally expected to do without any complaint. But I do have some good news for you. The fact that you haven't succumbed to the feeling of wanting to give up means your strength and your willpower are even greater. Do not be mistaken, you shouldn't have to power through and force yourself to continue working when you feel like giving up. Sometimes, we don't want to be strong women. And that's all right, but let's not forget that we *are* strong women.

With all the emotional distress that we may experience from burnout, let us not forget the physical manifestations as well. Our body doesn't function in multiple separate ways. Instead, everything is intertwining and interwoven, so when you experience emotional stress, it is guaranteed to show physically in some way or the other. Often, the first physical sign of burnout is fatigue and exhaustion. But this is a tricky one to pick up on because when we are so rooted in routine, the slightest change can leave us feeling sluggish and tired. But fatigue on its own is characterized by extreme tiredness and goes on for far longer than just that one night that you stayed up watching your favorite series. Fatigue and exhaustion becomes a prolonged problem when it starts affecting your daily functioning, and this, in turn, will cause a further lack of motivation, low confidence, and feeling dreadful toward your job.

The tricky thing about burnout and its physical manifestations is that it creates what may feel like a cycle. Burnout causes you to have a low immune system, you feel weak and tired, and you may experience excessive body aches, especially in the areas of your body that carry the most tension, such as your neck and upper shoulder. But because of your weakened immune system, you will find yourself getting sick and experiencing these symptoms all over again. What that means is that you may suffer from chronic muscle aches and body pains, and no amount of full-body Swedish massages will help, as those may just be temporary solutions.

Additionally, in experiencing fatigue and exhaustion, you may find difficulty in falling asleep. A lot of the time, this is because your mind is racing in anticipation, or dread, of what is to come the next day when you have to go back into the office and do a job that gives you anxiety. Yet another cycle is present—one of being completely tired but having the inability to sleep, making things worse and worse and harder and harder as it goes on.

As your sleep and your all-round emotional and physical health seems to deteriorate, this is only made worse as your appetite also seems to slowly disappear. Whether it is because your job is keeping you too occupied to eat, you find yourself unable to enjoy a wonderful meal, or you find yourself unable to eat anything that may be good for your body, not putting the right things into your body makes your output below par.

While there are many mental, physical, and emotional symptoms that one may experience from burnout, it has officially been classified as a syndrome. This means that each person may experience different combinations of symptoms related to burnout. This can sometimes even make it harder to pinpoint that you are experiencing burnout. While some people experience intense anxiety, others may be tired all the time, and others may experience combinations of these symptoms. But there are behavioral elements associated with burnout as well. In extreme cases, people may find themselves dabbling in drugs or alcohol to ease the pressure; they may find themselves absconding from work as a way of avoiding a place they don't want to go; and they may find themselves isolating from others and even avoiding responsibilities of work and life. But there are other more subtle behavioral elements to burnout. For example, when you come home and you feel touched out but your child is begging for attention, you may find yourself yelling for an entirely unwarranted reason. This adds to the overwhelming emotions that you're already feeling, and you find yourself feeling guilty because you yelled.

## The Difference Between Burnout and Stress

Remember the stress cycle we spoke about before? Our stress cycles either need to be completed or mitigated and resolved at one of its stages. Burnout is often a result of unresolved, continuous, and prolonged stress that never gets mitigated or concluded. So while the line between stress and burnout is often not very clear, there are some defining factors.

First, you can have stress without burnout, but you can't have burnout without stress. Burnout comes as a result of stress that goes on and on. This is either because you are not completing your stress cycle or your stress is not getting resolved at any point in the cycle.

Second, stress, as I mentioned before, is triggered as a safety mechanism. This means that once we perceive the threat to be over, we slowly come out of our stress cycle. This means that we know there is an end to the stress we may be experiencing, but with burnout, it seems like there is no end in sight. And it is from here that the extreme sense of dread stems.

Third, stress may motivate us to work faster; we may be frantic, but we always finish the task at hand. Being burnt out, on the other hand, makes you feel entirely withdrawn and not even prompted to try working on anything.

Last, when you are experiencing stress, you may feel the need to seek out professional help in the form of therapy. When you're burnt out, you don't even want to consider seeking help, and you may slip deeper and deeper into depression.

While stress is almost a guarantee, it is important to know your body's own stress signs so you don't find yourself falling into burnout.

# Chapter 3

# Getting to Know Your Body and Mind

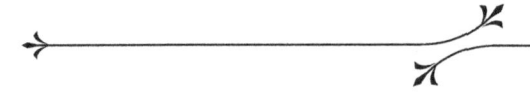

The human body is such an amazing and wonderful thing. It is fascinating the way the intricacies of everyday life are so interlinked, that our internal functions communicate, as if by magic, and that it is how we respond externally. The fact that we have a stress response that is designed to keep us alive and help us survive makes me step back and admire the human body in absolute awe. It is this awe that inspired me to pursue a career in health care. Something that further amazes me is how two people can react to the same occurrence in vastly different ways. This, for me, is absolutely mind-blowing.

Just in the same way that we would all react to one occurrence in different ways, we all react differently to stress and ultimately burnout. This, to some extent, makes treating stress and burnout far harder. Because of its lack of a one-size-fits-all approach, when speaking out about what you are feeling and seeking help, burnout may often be misdiagnosed. Everyone acts in a broadly different way, and that makes treating these different symptoms and finding a resolution a lot harder.

So how would we fix this? We would need to get back in touch with our bodies.

I know this may seem like a weird concept to think of because you're the one that is actually living in your body. You're really the only person in the world who knows what you are feeling and why. But as strange as it may sound, we do lose touch with ourselves and our bodies. It's almost as if we start going through the motions of life, totally oblivious and numb to the routine of everyday life. It is almost like we're on autopilot mode. Do you know the feeling of driving home from work, and before you know it, you're pulling up into the driveway completely unaware of the entire drive you just had? That's the feeling of being on autopilot.

Being out of touch with oneself can stem from many things, but one of the most common causes can be from this constantly crazy life that you may lead. Let me give you an example: Let us imagine that you have a job that has multiple deadlines and your schedule is often filled with back-to-back meetings that take away from the available time you have to complete these projects. When you come home, you have kids to take care of, dinner to prepare, a kitchen to clean, and so much more, even after a long commute from work to home.

Knowing the endless list of tasks that you have waiting for you may be enough to make you shut down. What pushes you more into autopilot mode is by knowing that, each day, the same routine follows. But this is why we have little things to look forward to, like vacations and weekends. But when your weekly routine spills into your weekend and you find yourself doing work when you're supposed to be refreshing yourself mentally, physically, and emotionally, this can lead to the constant stress growing greater and greater with each day.

Being out of touch with yourself can feel like you're going crazy because your head is so full with the to-do list you have to get through. You may even find yourself feeling overwhelmed by emotions, asking yourself what I have asked myself so often too: "Why do I feel this way?"

But if you feel disconnected and out of touch with yourself, there are many ways for you to "find yourself" once more. Some simple tips that you may come across will be to take time away from the routine. Yes, as humans, we thrive on routine, but sometimes it can blur the lines between one day and the next. Taking time away from your routine can mean stepping away from your computer by using some of those vacation days you're hesitant about using. It can mean something so simple as ending your week on the weekend, rather than just carrying on with more of the same. It can mean taking a long walk in the park, in your garden, or even down the street, which is especially beneficial if it isn't something you do very often. You can also reconnect with yourself through yoga and meditation or even just by being entirely alone with yourself.

I remember a really stressful time in my life where it felt like the only two roles I played were a mom and a worker. I had not only fallen out of touch with myself but with my partner too. That is until I gave myself the opportunity to get to know myself again. I took myself out for coffee, alone, and I tried to learn who I was again. It was successful, and my partner was really happy to learn who I was all over again too.

There are other ways, on a physiological level, where we lose touch with ourselves, and in turn, this may begin to affect our health. One such way is when we get so busy and hung up by the stresses of life that we begin letting things such as eating a healthy meal slide by. I have seen people so occupied with everyday life that they fail to do something as simple as eating their lunch. For these people, lunch often consists of quick snacks that aren't healthy and that are bad for their teeth, making my job as their dental provider a lot harder. After some time, their health begins to deteriorate, and they begin suffering from symptoms of low blood sugar and other symptoms that were a result of skipping meals. Skipping meals was only a by-product of the stress, but that by-product created further health issues.

While getting back in touch with your body can be as straightforward as doing things such as eating better, getting some exercise, and getting a good night's sleep, beyond that, it allows you to communicate better with your body. Now, you may be wondering what this communication does for stress and what its relation is to stress. If you know your body and you know what your stress triggers and first symptoms of stress are, you can begin implementing ways of mitigating your stress response before it escalates into burnout. Have you ever heard someone say, "I have a cold sore," or, "My hair has been falling out so much lately"? They usually follow this up by saying that it must be stress, or if they aren't saying it, someone else is telling them that it could probably be attributed to stress. But you are the only person who knows your body better than anyone. If you give yourself enough attention, focus on the little things, and begin communicating with your body, you will quickly realize your early warning signs for stress, and you will know when your body is in the midst of a stress cycle.

Personally, it took me a long time to reconnect with myself and figure out my own stress cycle and my own personal stress exhibitions. I found myself being extremely snappy and removed from those around me when I was under stress. It was only when I began getting more in touch with myself that I noticed when I would lash out and when I would feel this way. I started paying even closer attention, and this allowed me to prepare in advance. I found myself experiencing the highest levels of stress when I was required to carry out specific aspects of my duties as a dental provider at a private practice. One such duty is the submission of predeterminations for procedures and treatments to insurance companies. In these submissions, I am required to motivate and explain to the insurance company why the patient would need a specific treatment in order for the insurance company to cover the payment of these procedures.

After motivating and nearly pleading with insurance companies to cover the needed procedures for my patients, I would receive a frustrating response from the company, providing me with an alternative procedure that was cheaper and would ultimately be ineffectual in the treatment of the patient's need. As an example, after an initial consultation with a patient, I would see that they require an implant. I would reach out to the insurance company, and they would try to push for a cheaper alternative treatment such as a metal partial or denture, which is replacing the damaged or missing teeth while the patient still has much of their own teeth remaining, and that is the treatment that they would approve.

This caused me extreme stress every time I had to make the call to the patient's insurance company. It meant mentally trying to prepare myself because I already knew that the chances of getting the response I was hoping for were minimal. At this point, even before I made the call, I was already carrying a heavy mental load with my stress response activated and fully forming the ball of anxiety in my chest. I knew that when I was on the phone call, I was going to be begging, at least that's what it felt like—begging and pleading to justify a treatment. This stress would be further increased by getting no help or understanding from the company and then having to explain to the patient the treatment they need and the treatment their insurance actually covers.

This source of stress is something that I pinpointed quite fast, and it is something that I had to devise mechanisms to cope with every time these calls to the insurance companies were made. As a way of trying to ease this stress, I would take a few deep breaths before making the phone calls, and I would try to do calming exercises immediately before and immediately after making these stressful phone calls. This allowed me to be the most confident version of myself in motivating for the best treatment for my patients. It also allowed me to be a calmer version of myself for the patients I was seeing after that very stressful moment.

Through a combination of different stress management strategies, I was able to better handle the situations that I really didn't enjoy carrying out. I was able to find a way to make sure my stress cycle didn't spiral out of control. Taking a better approach to these stressful situations also helped me be a less-stressed version of myself when I got home to my family.

The thing about stress is that it usually doesn't happen in an instant. It happens so gradually and so slowly that you barely notice that you're in over your head until you really begin introspecting what is happening in your life. Because this change happens in an unnoticeable way, we usually only become aware of it when someone else points it out to us. It is at this point where we first take offense, and then we realize that we are actually going through some sort of physiological reaction. Whether we understand the intricacies of this change or not, all we know is that we have been removed from our most natural and most comfortable state, and now, we face a discomfort that we need to rectify.

## Physical Changes Caused by Fight-or-Flight

# Response

Although, as previously mentioned, the fight-or-flight response takes place on a physiological and unseen level, it does manifest in physical forms. These physical forms are what get us into action so we can respond appropriately to the perceived threat. We need to be able to recognize our own unique physical responses to stress, and we need to understand why it is important to recognize our responses. Let us look at the latter first. When you understand the physical manifestations of stress, you are able to not only recognize that you are stressed, but you're able to mitigate the stress response before it spirals out of control. Stress that has been left unchecked is what turns into burnout. If you identify that you are being stressed out by a specific event, task, or person, you can remove yourself from that situation or find the best possible way of making sure that stress doesn't get to you.

Now that we know why it's important, know what our triggers are, and recognize when we are in a stress cycle, we can begin looking at the physical manifestations of being stressed out. While the beginning stages of the stress cycle occur on a physiological level, as soon as it becomes physical, we need to be aware and alert to the changes that are taking place. Our bodies will experience a distinct change. From feeling a knot in your stomach and a lump in your throat, you may begin feeling other things such as a cold sweat spreading throughout your body, your heart rate quickening or your muscles trembling and shaking. However, when the stress cycle becomes prolonged and it is headed toward the road of burnout, you may begin experiencing difficulty sleeping or extreme exhaustion; you may find your body feeling out of sorts, whether it is achy or just all-around uncomfortable; you will have prolonged muscle tension and even your hands shaking, and you may begin feeling the overworking of your mind through headaches and dizziness.

These are many of the "well-known" symptoms of stress, but what about the other lesser known ones, the ones that eat into your productive time, without you even knowing about it? When I was younger and I was getting ready to go for my driver's test and get my license, I was very nervous, as are most people for such a momentous time in their life. But in the days leading up to my test, I found myself sleeping excessively. This was a strange manifestation of stress and anxiety, and I didn't even know that was the cause of it. After completing the test successfully, I came home and slept again. I realized that it was out of character and unlike me to be using my productive time to sleep, but the sheer exhaustion did not manifest itself in the form of yawning and tiredness; rather, it manifested as a deep need for sleep. It wasn't until I began writing finals and the same symptom of sleep presented itself that I realized the excessive sleeping was a result of stress.

Figuring out your unique symptom may take some keen observation before you pinpoint it. Perhaps the way you can stop or assist yourself during a stress cycle is by getting help, enforcing a deep meditation regimen, or doing yoga. When you know what your stressors are, you can then use tactics to calm your body that are directly targeted at that response. For example, when you are stressed, you find that your overall heart rate has increased. A good coping mechanism would be to begin purposeful and diaphragmatic breathing as a way to slow your heart rate. While breathing, you can focus on yourself and lay out the tasks you are hoping to complete in small steps and increments, which may help in your overall stress reduction.

As strange and fascinating as the concept of the internal processes of stress and the fight-or-flight mechanism may be, the curiosity and focus go far deeper than that. Since stress and burnout have become such a focal point in recent years, people have found themselves wondering if there are certain people that are more susceptible to burnout than others. Two things that have presented themselves as answers to this question are the idea of personality types and professions. On a less influential level are general circumstances, and recently, stress and burnout overall have been heightened as a result of the global COVID-19 pandemic. At the onset of the pandemic, people were extremely stressed even about leaving their homes, but tossed into all of that was learning how to work from home, how to homeschool their kids, and how to manage the new stress of a pandemic and the stress of the rising costs and a dropping economy. But these circumstances, although few and far between, affected the entire world.

If we look first at professions, it has been seen that a caregiver career tends to face burnout more often and faces the highest rates of burnout than others. People in caregiving roles such as doctors and nurses and people who find themselves working in jobs that they are extremely passionate about may find themselves more burnt out than in other professions. This is because they may find it harder to draw the line between what they love doing and what their job is. Because they are working in passion-driven jobs and they are caring for others, they may not know when to step away and take care of themselves. Because of this burnout, it has also been found that suicide rates are higher for people who are in passion-driven and caregiver positions (Moss, 2019).

In addition to the type of profession that causes burnout, there are also certain personality types that are more likely and susceptible to experience burnout than others. We all know of someone in our lives that seems constantly high-strung, someone who's easily spooked, and someone who seems like they are constantly anxious. The following are some of the personality traits that put people at a higher risk of experiencing burnout (Scott, 2020):

- Being a perfectionist. While it is one thing to want to gain high achievements and strive to be the best that you are, perfectionists tend to be extremely hard on themselves if things are anything less than the utmost best. Yes, you can aspire for greatness and be happy if you get close to your goals, but a perfectionist will not be happy with anything that isn't perfect, even if their own capabilities allow them to achieve perfection.
- Being a pessimist. You have probably heard of the glass-half-full or glass-half-empty analogy more times than you care to admit, but a pessimist is very likely to view the world in an overall more negative way than an optimist. They may experience everything as a threat or as potentially harmful, or when purposefully looking for the risks in something, they entirely avoid the potential benefits. Because of this constant negativity, they may be more likely to experience burnout.
- Being overly excitable. As previously mentioned, we all know someone who is constantly high-strung. But we also know someone who is easily triggered and is set off by the smallest thing. We all know

someone who we somewhat have to tiptoe around because we don't know what may set them off. These people are more likely to experience stress and mental overload that comes with a job, and they are more likely to experience burnout.

- Being extremely doubtful and unfit for the job. There are those who thrive on positive feedback, then there are those who suffer from severe imposter syndrome and who think they are just not good enough for the role they have. This makes them try to put in more effort even though they are exceeding just as they are. There are also people who are unfit for their roles. I, for one, am extremely aware of my abilities, and I know that I will never succeed as a sales associate. If I were placed in such a position, all of the elements of my role and my job would result in me being unsuccessful despite working hard, which in turn will lead to burnout.

- Having a type A personality. Whether this is a term you are familiar with or not, type A is a personality type that is highly driven and work-oriented; they are aggressive in their work approaches and aim to meet goals quite aggressively. Type A is focused on the final result, whereas type B personalities find themselves more laid back and focused on the journey rather than the destination. While type A personalities are the people most employers hope to have on their team, they are more likely to experience burnout from their excessively

aggressive approach to work and their susceptibility to heart illness.
- This shows that burnout can be triggered by internal and external factors.

## The Idea of Syndrome

As previously mentioned, each person experiences the symptoms of stress and burnout in different ways. While there is a general list of symptoms that people experience when they are highly stressed out or on the verge of being burnt out or entirely burnt out, some people may never experience these stipulated symptoms and may experience symptoms that could be entirely new to the list of identifying factors of stress.

By virtue of stress and burnout causing different manifestations in different people, it has therefore been classified as a syndrome (Jones, 2017).

As a dental professional, one of the symptoms that I actively see in my patients when they suffer from severe stress or burnout is the traces of bruxism. Bruxism is the medical term that refers to the grinding of one's teeth and the clenching of one's jaw that happens frequently and usually while you are unaware. Bruxism can be caused by a number of factors, including stress, and is associated with someone who has a type A personality. It has also been found that people who experience severe anger and frustration may experience bruxism (Johns Hopkins Medicine, 2021).

As a dentist, I have seen the signs of bruxism clearly in a number of my patients, and once I get to talk with them, I realize that it stems from a real place of stress, anxiety, frustration, and even burnout. While bruxism can also be caused by antidepressants and an imbalance of neurotransmitters, this further goes to show that certain symptoms may reflect multiple syndromes.

Bruxism is easy enough for me as a dental provider to identify. I see things such as abrasions to the teeth, marks on the tongue, and scarring on the inside of my patients' cheeks. I also see flattened tips of the teeth, eroded enamel, and strain or clicking on my patients' jaws. But as a healthcare professional, I know what I am looking for.

How would you, as a sufferer of bruxism, know what to look out for? Bruxism comes with multiple side effects. You may find yourself experiencing intense headaches, especially on the sides and temple areas of your head. Because your teeth are being clenched tightly together, tension begins forming in your head and can easily lead to intense headaches. Sometimes, you're only made aware of it when someone asks you to unclench your jaw. Bruxism is so subtle that it even happens in your sleep. My son experienced bruxism in his sleep as a young child which only occurred when he was teething. He was not under any form of stress, and yet he would grind his teeth constantly.

There are other ways of knowing if you suffer from bruxism, and that is by feeling numbness or pain in your face and facial muscles; you find yourself with chipped or broken teeth, or you notice a clicking sound on your jaw that is accompanied by a lockjaw or a dislocation of your jaw. But the thing about bruxism is that a lot of these symptoms may be related to other systemic problems as well. It is for this reason that if you experience any of these signs, it is imperative that you do not try to self-diagnose and that you seek medical help and attention.

There are multiple treatments available for bruxism depending on your age, if it is related to stress or to another health condition, and if you are eligible to take certain medications. Once this has been established, you may be taught certain mechanisms to employ that will help you relax your jaw, face, and tongue; you could be prescribed medications, physical therapy; or you will be issued with a mouthguard to prevent grinding from continuing.

Whether it is from stress or not, bruxism is caused by serious concerns that should implore you to see your dentist or doctor if you notice any symptoms.

# Chapter 4

# Finding Your Coping Mechanism

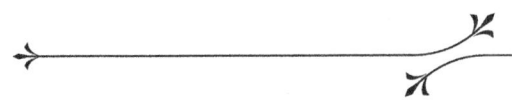

There have been countless times where I have heard even nonsmokers look upon their work with extreme distress and say that they need a cigarette. Yes, it may just have been a joke, but the relationship between stress and smoking is one that we are all familiar with.

From a very young age, we are offered assistance when we are in distress. As a baby, we are offered a pacifier as a way of soothing ourselves; we use it as a comfort and a way of taking our mind off something that we are unhappy about. This becomes a coping mechanism for us to deal with, and handle stressful situations. But a lot of the time, this coping mechanism can be negative. As a dentist, I have seen many young children come in who suck their thumb or are dependent on a pacifier to cope and soothe themselves, and it often leads to improper development in the structure of the mouth and misalignment of the teeth.

Ultimately, through the negative effects that a pacifier has on a child's development, it may be classified as a negative coping mechanism. But before we can even find a coping mechanism that suits us or before we are able to differentiate between positive and negative coping mechanisms, we need to know what a coping mechanism is. A coping mechanism is something that we use to cope with stress or a traumatic event; it helps us deal with emotional changes, whether it is the everyday stresses that we face or coping with an immediate and dramatic change (GoodTherapy, 2018). Coping mechanisms are great for helping you manage the stress of your day-to-day jobs and getting through work and the duties that you need to fulfill at home. But even beyond that, coping mechanisms can help you cope with the loss of a loved one; it can help you cope if you face an incident such as getting robbed or even losing your job.

People can experience negative stress, as well as positive stress. Yes, you may need to find ways to cope with death, loss, and fear, but even good and momentous life events can cause us stress. Think about a big day that you are extremely excited about. It could be a function or a birthday event that you are throwing; it could be the expected birth of your baby or of a close relative's baby; it could be the excitement of a graduation, or it could be a wedding that you're excited about. Although not negative, these positive events also place your body under some form of stress (GoodTherapy, 2018).

As time progresses and as our lives progress, we are always presented with some form of stress. It is something that has existed since the dawn of time, and it is something that will exist for years still to come. While there are many uncertainties, one thing is certain, and that is that, as humans, we will always be exposed to stressful situations, and it is up to us to handle those situations in a healthy way.

Just in the same way that we all experience stress differently, we all develop different coping mechanisms that best get us through the situations we face. For some, these coping mechanisms are behavioral, whereby they may find themselves going for a walk outside, listening to music, taking themselves out for dinner and coffee, or taking on some sort of physical activity like yoga or jogging. But people may also have different coping mechanisms for different situations. For example, if a person experiences work stress, they may cope by listening to classical music in the background while they work, whereas dealing with a divorce or an argument with their partner may lead to them consuming large amounts of junk food. As unique as the person and the stress is, that's how unique the coping mechanism will be.

But how do you know if a particular coping mechanism is good for you, if it works for you, and if it is healthy? The thing about coping mechanisms is that they can be bad for us. A lot of the time, people have very addictive personalities, and if the thing they use to cope with stress is addictive, it can often lead them down a destructive path. I once read somewhere that pleasure does not define happiness, and often in the pursuit of pleasure, we are led down destructive paths because we confuse the fleeting, temporary feeling of pleasure with happiness. But coping mechanisms are not necessarily meant to be pleasurable. Now, this does not mean that you can't gain some sort of joy from your coping mechanisms, but ultimately, your coping mechanism is not going to remove the stressor from your life. Rather, it will make the stress more bearable. It will equip you to maintain your composure and your internal balance despite being in a stressful situation. These mechanisms allow you to acknowledge that you are in a stressful situation, but it helps you maintain composure and a good headspace that does not lead to detrimental aftereffects.

There are two types of coping mechanisms that exist, namely, active and avoidant. Active coping mechanisms refer to knowing and understanding that you are under stress but using tactics to actively attempt to reduce your stress (GoodTherapy, 2018). This can mean rationalizing your thoughts, explaining to yourself why you are not in immediate danger or establishing means and methods to overcome the situation that is presenting the stress, whether it is employing immediate breathing exercises or closing your eyes and just focusing on some constants in your space. The next type of coping mechanism is known as the avoidant mechanism whereby you try to ignore or avoid the stressor at all costs. This is not a viable or long-term solution to stress because if you are triggered by something like traffic, for example, it will be hard for you to continue functioning if you try to avoid traffic (GoodTherapy, 2018).

However, over and above active and avoidant coping mechanisms, people may employ the use of different items or behavioral tactics to manage their stress which may be negative. Some of these mechanisms provide the temporary pleasure that distracts from the stress but does not actively aid in mitigating the stress you are experiencing. It is similar to putting a Band-Aid on a gunshot wound. In the long run, these coping mechanisms can be negative.

A coping mechanism can be negative when a person employs things such as drugs, cigarettes, alcohol, and other precarious behaviors that could cause more harm than good. The thing about these negative coping mechanisms is that it numbs the feeling of stress and frustration only temporarily, but once it wears off, the stress comes flooding back, often more severe than it was before because it wasn't addressed in any direct way before. This is where an addiction cycle comes in, and it is developed in one of two ways. The first is that once the effects of these coping mechanisms wear off, the stress comes back even more severe than before, which leads to a person trying to reintroduce the same level of relief that they previously experienced. Every time the stress resurfaces, they turn to alcohol or drugs or whatever it is they are using to help the intense feelings of stress, and because the stress is never addressed at the source, it is almost guaranteed to resurface, and they are required to keep on using these substances to cope. They become dependent on it to ease their anxiety and frustration.

The second is that a lot of substances or coping mechanisms have addictive traits, and as previously mentioned, people may have addictive personalities. Things such as food, drugs, alcohol, cigarettes, and other behaviors actually result in addiction. People either get addicted to the elements within the substance, for example, some drugs and cigarettes contain substances that are extremely addictive, or they may also get addicted to the feeling and sensation that they feel when they engage in the use of these substances.

People may enjoy the feeling of having certain drugs; they may enjoy the feeling and the sensation they experience when they take in high volumes of alcohol, or they may even just enjoy the night's sleep they experience afterward. I have had a lot of patients come in to see me, and they openly say that they don't like smoking, they don't like the smell of cigarette smoke, or they don't enjoy being around other smokers, but they are addicted to the nicotine in the tobacco.

In these cases, coping mechanisms can be extremely negative, because in all instances they cause harm and they don't directly help in mitigating the stress or the stressor. As an example, if you are completely stressed out about an upcoming deadline and you begin smoking as a way to deal with the stress, you are creating an addiction for yourself without actually taking action to resolve the stress and implementing processes to meet the deadline effectively. This is a negative coping mechanism.

Alternatively, a positive coping mechanism would be creating a to-do list to tackle the tasks within the project one by one in a stipulated time frame. This will make it easier to complete smaller chunks of the project rather than expecting yourself to take on a whole project in one tight deadline. You may find yourself looking for time management tactics to help yourself deal with each part of the project, or you may even find yourself taking a leap to communicate with those around you to manage expectations in completing the project and requesting ways and means of adjusting the deadline. These are positive coping mechanisms in that they help you take on the stress directly.

## Finding Positive Coping Mechanisms

Ultimately, we try to use coping mechanisms through cognitive or behavioral means, to help us either remove, reduce, or prevent stress from occurring. There are multiple types of coping mechanisms that you can employ that will assist you with the different types of stressors you may face.

The first type of coping strategy, which was briefly discussed above, is problem-focused mechanisms. These are the mechanisms that address the cause of the stress directly. This is the way you would devise and implement strategies to directly resolve the issue that is causing your stress, such as figuring out ways to meet a looming work deadline that is making you nervous (Dreamcloud Editorial Team, 2019).

The next type is emotional-focused mechanisms. While these coping mechanisms do not directly work toward mitigating the source of the stress, they are personal and help you to personally deal with the stress.

However, this strategy can both tip toward being negative or positive. Some people may find themselves taking in negative emotions as a way of trying to cope; they may begin complaining excessively, shutting themselves off from those around them, or even crying. But there are positive ways of utilizing emotional-focused mechanisms. Perhaps you may find yourself turning to a spiritual higher power in the pursuit of emotional relief. You may look for social support by speaking to others or asking for help from someone around you or even seeking out therapy which is also a form of social coping. Through social coping, you may find yourself off-loading a mental load and talking to others to relieve the stress you may be feeling. You may even find solace in turning to humor as a way of coping with stress (Dreamcloud Editorial Team, 2019).

The next type of coping mechanism is the meaning-focused mechanism. This is where you search, introspectively, about why you may be stressed out and you search internally for solutions to the root cause of the stress or rather your reaction to the stress. You may find yourself asking why you are triggered by the stress and why you are feeling stressed out by a particular situation, and you find yourself looking for ways to strengthen yourself and build resilience toward the stressors (Dreamcloud Editorial Team, 2019).

For each type of coping strategy, there are healthy and unhealthy mechanisms. For you to find the one that best suits you, you will need to identify your triggers and what the greatest causes of stress are in your life. If you find that you are more of an emotional person and you seek to deal with stress through emotional-focused coping mechanisms, there are a number of great tactics that you can use to reduce stress. The first would be journaling and writing down your thoughts and emotions. This usually makes it easier to come back later when you experience the same feelings and find ways of making yourself feel better. You can also utilize tactics such as yoga and meditation to calm yourself and your feelings from the inside.

While these focus on the internal and emotional ways of coping with stress, you may find it becoming a daily practice that eases you into facing any curveball that life may throw at you. On the flip side of that same coin, you may find yourself tackling the stressor head-on, making to-do lists, and planning ahead of time. You may not find your coping mechanism the first time around, and you may need to try a few methods before you find one that works for you. But when you do find one that works for you repeatedly, you can continue using this healthy coping mechanism for all the stress that life may throw at you.

## Finding the Relaxation

Coping with stress and employing the best coping mechanisms play an important role in your stress cycle.

It helps you ride the highs and lows with the best possible steps in place to ensure that your stress cycle is completed, isn't interrupted midway, and does not persist for long periods of time leading to burnout. Not only that, if you find something that works as a coping mechanism that is feasible, and that you really enjoy doing, you may find yourself encountering a new hobby. I have a dear friend who, in the midst of her daily stresses caused by her job, began seeking a creative outlet and a creative mechanism for stress relief. She dabbled in music and found that learning a new instrument seemed to be too stressful in its own right; she learned that drawing was not her niche, and she found way too much stress and pressure in perfecting her drawing pieces, and then she tried her hand at painting. She was an absolute natural. She found so much peace in painting, and it turned out to be one of her favorite pastimes. What's more, she began getting commissions and eventually left her job to dedicate all of her time to painting.

It is important to remember however that you do not need to experience burnout to know what to avoid in the future. Some people push themselves so hard and their response is that they have never been burnt out before, so chances are it won't happen. No. That is not the way anyone should live their life. When our cars are giving us trouble or they are due for their annual maintenance, we take them off the road immediately and make sure it is taken great care of. We won't keep it on the road for fear of meeting with an accident. So why would we push our bodies, for which there are no spare parts available when it is telling us to take it a bit easier?

Something that I respond to within these instances is that if you have never experienced burnout before, how do you know you are not experiencing it now? Do you want to test your limits enough so that when you do get burnt out you can say, "Ah, yes, that was too much, and that is when I need to stop," or would you rather make sure that you never have to go through that ever? My philosophy is that prevention is better than cure.

To find coping mechanisms that will work for you, you will need to find a task or an activity that you can do to relax. I know that it often seems like relaxation is out of reach or maybe you have an unrealistic expectation of relaxation, but it doesn't always need to be a full body massage or looking out at a sunset over a lake when you live nowhere near a lake. Relaxation can come in many ways, shapes, and forms. Relaxation also doesn't mean taking time away from your desk or computer but still talking and thinking about work. When you go forward with the aim of relaxing, you need to make sure that you try to be as fully present at the moment as you can be. So if you decide to go for a walk with your family as your time of physical relaxation, you need to try and make sure that you are not thinking or talking about work. This is going to be difficult to do at first, but through conscious effort, you will find yourself more aware of where you are and what should be filtering through into that space.

Once you establish boundaries for yourself and your "sacred" space of relaxation, you can then begin finding the best forms of relaxation for yourself. We have already seen that stress and burnout have physical manifestations on your body. So let us begin by looking at physical relaxation techniques. When you are stressed out, your body begins holding onto tension in certain parts. This may make your neck feel sore, your shoulders ache, or your head hurt. But physical relaxation techniques have been proven to ease stiffness in your body and lower your cortisol levels.

The first method of physical relaxation that you can use is breathing exercises. Breathing forms the most fundamental element of human survival, but when used on a deeper level, it can reduce stress and frustration. Have you noticed that when you're stressed, panicked, or under severe strain, you feel like you can't catch your breath? Many people, when experiencing an anxiety attack, may begin hyperventilating. This response is enough to show our bodies that the best way to counter such an attack would be to make efforts to focus on our breathing. Perhaps breathing is such a natural occurrence that, when we are overly stressed out, we even forget to breathe. But there are a number of breathing techniques that can be used to reduce stress and find relaxation. It is recommended that, first, you place yourself in a comfortable position, either standing, sitting on a chair, or lying on your back with your palms facing upward. You are then going to focus on your breathing and start by taking a deep breath in while counting to five, and then immediately release the breath while counting to five again. It is recommended that you breathe in through your nose and out through your mouth. It is also recommended that you repeat this entire process for about three to five minutes (NHS, 2021).

Breathing exercises, along with other techniques that will be discussed below, form part of the relaxation response. Now, we have heard of the stress cycle and the stress response, and after all of that heavy information, hearing the words relaxation response may be somewhat of a breath of fresh air. The relaxation response is not some exotic massage that will cost you a fortune. Instead, it is a way of basically counteracting your body's stress response system, and it is basically the opposite of your fight-or-flight response. The relaxation response is part of the parasympathetic nervous system which is the rest and digest process of your body. It is the part that is shut down when your body experiences danger and your fight-or-flight response is activated (Scott, 2019).

When you are experiencing high levels of stress, you can reverse the release of cortisol by activating the relaxation response through a number of methods, the first of which was discussed above through purposeful breathing. The next way of inducing your relaxation response is through meditation. It has become almost universally known that during meditation, leaders would encourage those around them to sit in a meditation pose and repeat the same sound over and over again. In most cases, the word "om" is chanted. While there are many different meditation methods, it always proves as a great way of reducing stress because it calms both the mind and the body (Scott, 2019).

The next method is progressive muscle relaxation. This technique of inducing the relaxation response requires a lot of concentration, which I am convinced contributes to one's ability to momentarily remove the stress from your mind. During this technique, you can tense certain muscles and then relax them in different areas of your body (Scott, 2019). When you are paying specific attention to relaxing your muscles, you become more aware of what was tense in the first place. In my own personal case, I often find the muscles of my face to be tense when I am under stress. My forehead will be creased, my brows will be pulled together, my lips will be taut, and I am usually biting my lip in frustration. But when I use progressive muscle relaxation, I tell myself to release my forehead, then my eyebrows, and then my mouth. While I am doing so, I usually find that my cheeks are tensed up too and that my ears are somehow taking strain as well. It is after that, that I become aware of what was tense and what was relaxed, and I consciously make an effort to relax myself.

Lastly, another great way of inducing your relaxation response is by doing exercise and yoga. Moving your body in its physical space releases endorphins and limits the release of cortisol. It is hard to stay stressed when your body is running on an amazing high.

Aside from the physical ways of inducing the relaxation response, there are other ways and means of becoming more relaxed. Sometimes, you may not be in a physical mood; perhaps you are more of a creative or analytical type of person rather than a physical person. In this instance, you may try using emotional and mental methods of attempting to achieve the bliss that comes with relaxation.

Aside from utilizing art forms and creative outlets as a means of expression and as a way to de-stress, other methods that may be beneficial in achieving the relaxation response are changing your own personal narrative and finding and engaging in some sort of spiritual practice. To some extent, these two elements go hand in hand. If you do believe in a higher power, you believe that through faith you have been created and that your Creator makes no mistake. If your Creator would not allow anyone to speak negatively of you, why should you be the one to speak negatively of yourself? However, you may either be spiritual or choose to change your narrative in two unrelated ways. First, getting in touch with a spiritual practice allows you to remember your greater purpose. It allows you to retrospectively glance back at your life and see that your circumstances are so minute in the greater scheme of things or that whatever you are facing and dealing with is exactly where you're meant to be and it is a stepping stone to a greater version of yourself. By changing your internal narrative, you remind yourself of the positive that you have not only done in the past but that you are also capable of achieving in the future.

Something that I have also found to be relaxing and just overall beneficial to myself is creating a gratitude list. When I was feeling at my worst and at my lowest, I would write a list of all the things I was grateful for and all the things I was lucky to have. I listed the big things like my family, my friends, my home, and my job, but I even listed the small things like the chocolate bar I was able to eat, my comfy pillow, and my lights turning on with literally a flick of a button. It allowed me to realize that others were not as fortunate as me and to just be grateful.

Other ways that can help you gain relaxation is by journaling and doing a brain dump to clear your mind of everything that may have accumulated over the day. Once you write all the things that were stressing you out, you need to remind yourself to forget those moments. It becomes the notepad's problem. Next, you can aim to take on an optimistic frame of mind and attempt to connect with people either who are experiencing the same thing as you or who are entirely different. And lastly, you can rationalize with yourself and ask yourself if you are generalizing, overreacting, or jumping to conclusions about what you are currently experiencing.

No one can level with you the way you can. In all honesty, you are the only person who can be honest with yourself. So question the negativity, ask yourself if you are being dramatic, and allow yourself to overcome what is bringing you down. But most importantly, *never* underestimate your ability to bounce back from a low point.

# Chapter 5

# Time Management Made Easy

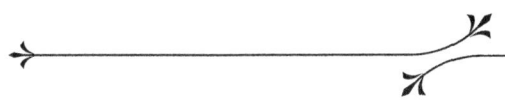

---

The concept of time management is one that seems to have always slipped out of my hands when I was the one in control of it. I found my time perfectly managed when I wasn't the one in charge of it. That is until I found myself suddenly in a position where I was the only one available to manage my time, and the stakes were high—the stakes included fetching my kids from school on time, attending parent-teacher meetings, and seeing a certain number of patients within a particular time. I felt like I was going to crash and burn, and that was when I realized that time management is the only way to thrive in life.

Time management allows you to give time, attention, and balance to the things that are most important to you while making sure that you also find some level of internal balance. Being a mom, a professional, a wife, and someone who takes a keen interest in her health, I used to find myself saying that society requires so much from women; there is no way that we'd find the time to do everything we're supposed to do in just 24 hours. As women, we're expected to work hard at our jobs, work hard at being a mother, do everything we can for our partner, keep our house looking phenomenal, take care of our health, and maintain healthy friendships, and we are expected to do all of this without asking for help because that may make you look weak. This seemed like too great a burden to carry, and that is when I noticed my health and fitness levels started slipping. But then I decided to better manage my time. Through better time management and the skills I am going to share with you; I managed to do all of these things and more in a decent amount of time.

Time management can be used in every facet of your life and is great for avoiding burnout because you give yourself downtime while ensuring you give yourself enough time to work and complete a specific task. While time management in itself may seem like an exhaustive task and may even feel like a waste of time, I am going to share with you seven steps on how you can get the most out of the 24 hours you have in a day.

When I found myself searching for time management techniques, there were a lot of long training exercises that gave me more stress rather than helped ease my stress. This is because I was running low on time, and it was a resource that I didn't have enough of to dedicate to making notes and lists or following instructions. But what I did come across were useful steps that quickly became second nature and became a part of my daily routine.

## Step One: Start by Setting Goals

Yes, we all have goals. We have all humbly practiced our responses to the question of where we see ourselves in five years, and we are consistently taking steps to try and meet those goals. But sometimes, goals need to be small for our own headspace and for our own stress levels. Sometimes, setting a goal can be as simple as saying you're not going to hit snooze on any of your alarms. Sometimes setting a goal can look like just getting out of your bed and making your bed. So it is important to note that before you even start setting goals, you define what a goal means to you. A goal is having an aim, an ambition, or the desired result that you are hoping to achieve. But the parameters of your goals need to be set by you. You need to decide how big or small your goal is going to be and how you're going to achieve it.

Something that I learned is that we need to set SMART goals. SMART is an acronym that stands for specific, measurable, attainable, realistic, and time-bound. The idea of setting SMART goals was created by George Doran, Arthur Miller, and James Cunningham in their 1981 article: "There's a S.M.A.R.T. way to write management goals and objectives." While the title of their article shows us that it was intended for management goals and objectives, many people have found the elements to be transferable into other facets of life, and it has quickly become the gold standard for the way people set goals in every area of their lives. But let us break it down even further (CFI Team, 2022):

Specific. When you are making your list of goals for your career or your job, it is important to make sure that your goals are specific. If they are specific, it makes it easier for you to accomplish because you are breaking it down for yourself in clear-cut instructions on how to achieve that goal. It is at this stage that you will include the five "W" questions. In the details of this step, you will include who will be included in helping you achieve this goal, where is the place that you will achieve your goal, what exactly you are hoping to achieve, when you would like to achieve this goal, and why do you want to achieve this goal.

Measurable. Your goals need to be measurable as a way of checking your progress. If there is nothing for you to measure yourself against, you will not be able to see how far you have come. I, personally, am someone who loves to see what I have achieved and how far I am when reaching my end goal. If your goal is not measurable, how would you know how far you've come and how much more you have left to go?

Attainable. Your goals need to be achievable. You can't hope to receive a promotion to C.E.O. when you are currently still on the market for a new job. You need to make sure that you are equipped with the resources that will help you achieve your goals.

Realistic. Your goal needs to be achievable in the time frame and in the manner that you hope to achieve them. Often, when we set unrealistic goals, we feel as though we have failed when we do not achieve them. But this is not a reflection on us but rather on our inability to set effective and realistic goals.

Timely. If you set a goal that has no deadline, you could achieve it tomorrow, or you could never achieve it. When something has a deadline attached to it, we work harder to achieve it. The time constraint serves as a motivation to complete your goal.

Setting a SMART goal is your way to success. But let us look at an example of how to set a SMART goal. If someone works in a corporate job and they are looking to grow in the company in the next year, their ultimate goal would be to obtain a promotion. Their SMART goal would look like this:

They would lay out specific structures and guidelines that they will use to achieve their goal. If they are hoping to move from an administrative role to a managerial role, they will first need to determine what they are hoping for. They are hoping for a title change and the benefits and compensation that would come with that title change. They are also hoping for more responsibility and more opportunities to prove themselves to those around them. Next, they would need to determine who would be involved in them achieving their goal. They would need to let their direct superior know they are hoping for a promotion and that they would like their performance reviewed. They will also need to depend on themselves to put in the work and the effort to achieve their goal.

Their goal would need to be measurable. They will need to state exactly what change they are hoping to achieve with this goal. Measurable would be hoping for greater monthly compensation, so in monetary value, there will be a measurement.

Their goal would need to be achievable. They cannot hope for a promotion in a department that they are not currently in, and they cannot hope for a promotion to a position for which they have no experience, expertise, or qualifications.

They would need to make sure that their goal is realistic; they cannot expect to go from an administrator to C.E.O. in one swift motion. They would need to follow the most natural order of development and growth within a company and take steps to move into the next position of growth that they are presented with.

Lastly, they would need to set a timeline for when they would hope to achieve this promotion and when they would like to carry out the smaller steps in obtaining the promotion. For example, perhaps they would need to present themselves to management, showing their performance. They would need to set a time when they would like to present to them. Maybe a realistic time for their performance to be reviewed and for the company policy to apply, they may need to set their goal for six months.

Once you have set out your SMART goals, you may feel extremely motivated and ready to conquer the world, but remember, this is just the first step of your seven-step time management strategy. The first step in handling your time is making sure that you have certain things you are hoping to achieve in the time you have. If you can't accomplish these goals in six months, for example, then you either have to adjust the time you are going to dedicate to achieving your goal (i.e., you are going to need to dedicate more time to the goal) or you are going to need to adjust the deadline for your goal (i.e., push the deadline out by a few weeks or months that would make it more realistic to achieve).

## Step Two: Make a To-Do List

Some people may say that they aren't "list" people. But I, for one, thrive on a to-do list, and I often cannot function if I haven't listed what I need to do for the day. Without a to-do list, my head feels as though it is extremely full and that something may fall out. For fear of forgetting to do something, a to-do list plays an integral role in me successfully completing the tasks I set out to achieve.

When talking to my friends and people close to me, I have often seen that those who steer away from a to-do list often don't know how to create a to-do list. Unfortunately, it is not as simplistic and useless as it may sound. Yes, a to-do list is as simple as doing a brain dump of everything you need to do and complete in the day, but in its completely raw form, it holds no structure and no accountability. Once you have done a rough form of your to-do list and thrown everything that you need to complete on paper, I then like to move on to a more detailed version of my list. If I have one task on my list, such as completing a writing project, I then break that down into smaller tasks. I will put, as subitems, things that I need to complete for that particular task. I will add the task of completing an outline, planning my resources, writing or typing the piece that I need to write, and then finally editing the project.

Once I have all my tasks and subtasks listed down, it makes it easier to visualize what I need to complete, which helps me not to underestimate the time it will take to complete the task. If I see one big task, it seems overwhelming, and I can't estimate how long it will take me to complete it. But breaking it down into smaller elements makes it easier.

Next, I reorganize my to-do list in terms of priority. At the top of my list, I put the most important item that may demand most of my time and focus. With that being at the top of the list, it is the first thing I see. I have also found myself avoiding tasks that seem difficult or that I just don't feel like doing. I avoid those items, I leave them for last, and I am too tired or mentally drained by the end of the day to attend to these tasks, which actually turn out to be quicker tasks that I just created a bad image of in my mind. As strange as it may sound, tasks that I do not look forward to doing are tasks that I also place at the top of my to-do list. This helps me get them out of the way without leaving them to be completed in a stress-induced state later on when it is due.

While I am more of a pen-and-paper kind of to-do list person, there are a number of digital tools that can assist you when completing tasks. You can use your calendar on your computer, laptop, or phone; you can use a downloaded application, or you may even use alarms to ring at certain times to keep you alert of what you should be working on. It is best to use whatever works for you, but it is also beneficial to ensure that no matter what tool you are using, your to-do list is visible to you at all times. This will help you see what you have completed, what you haven't completed as yet, and how you are doing in terms of the time you have to complete a task.

It may also be extremely helpful for you to create different to-do lists for different aspects of your life. If you have one for work, it can stay on your work desk. You can then also have one for your home where you list the tasks you would need to complete when you're at home. These may be tasks that don't happen every day or as part of your daily routine but that need to be completed before a certain deadline, such as helping your child with a school project, attending a parent-teacher meeting, or preparing dinner if you're having guests come over at your home.

If you're wondering what your to-do list should look like, you should know that it is not guaranteed to be some excessively or overly Pinterest-worthy picture of cute planners, washi tapes, and colored and glitter pens. On some days, your to-do list may be a scrap piece of paper with rough scribbles on it and scratches and reordering and readjusting. And that is fine. As long as you understand it and it helps you get your tasks done, that is all that matters. However, if you are looking for a more structured approach, you could always find detailed organizers at your local stationery store, or you could download a free template. A template may be structured in a list format with a checkbox to tick off if you have completed the item and another checkbox that will state the priority of the task. You can create your own specific key that tells you what is the most important and what is the least important. You can list the items from one to five, with one being the priority and five being the least important; you could use colors or you could use numbers. Once again, as long as you understand it, that is what is most important.

## Step Three: Focus on Results

Being result-driven is a great way of staying motivated. Have you ever noticed how hard it is to first start working out, but as soon as you see that you have lost some pounds on the scale or some inches off your waist, you're immediately motivated to work harder? That is because results are like positive reinforcements. It shows you that what you have been doing works, and it encourages you to continue doing it.

Sticking to timelines and time-managed tasks may help you see results but only if done correctly. Remember that this whole process is not the same fix for everyone but rather finding a solution that works best for you. It may take some readjusting of your time and how you have structured your tasks before you actually see results, but take some time to do trial runs where you assess whether a certain schedule is realistically going to work for you or not.

When you do eventually see results, you will know that it has been worth the effort and worth the time.

## Step Four: Have a Lunch Break

I know this sounds weird; after all, how strange it is that you have to be reminded to eat food, but sometimes, when you are so busy, so stressed, and so overwhelmed and on the verge of being burnt out, you forget the little things like eating, taking bathroom breaks, and going to bed at a reasonable time. But taking breaks and eating is extremely important.

For me, having lunch is a great way of stepping away from the tasks at hand and giving myself some mental space. I am rejuvenating my mind, but I am also feeding my body, which is important to remain fully functional. Often, taking care of ourselves falls to the bottom of the priority list while we fumble through trying to get things done that are actually important or, at least, appear more important than we actually are. We are also currently living in a world where basic human hygiene and basic human needs are considered alone time or self-care. I have seen many mothers come in to bring their kids for their dentist appointments, and these moms, who work full-time jobs, are extremely exhausted. When they are working, they are constantly working, and when they are at home, they are constantly needed, so much so that for them, going to the bathroom or taking a five-minute shower, or even having a quick snack is considered peace or a luxury.

Having a snack or lunch is important to step away and refresh yourself.

## Step Five: Prioritize Important Tasks

If this hasn't already been reiterated enough, it is extremely important to prioritize which tasks are important and which are less important and which tasks are probably fine being left for tomorrow. When we are working our way through tasks, we get confused between tasks that are considered urgent and tasks that are considered important. Former U.S. President Dwight D. Eisenhower postulated the Eisenhower's Principle, which states that there is a clear and distinct line between tasks that are important and tasks that are urgent. It is through this principle that Eisenhower established the importance of not just being efficient with time management but also being effective with your time (Mind Tools Content Team, n.d.).

Important tasks are defined as those that are pertinent to us achieving our own goals. The completion of these tasks holds great value to us personally.

However, on the other hand, urgent tasks are not important but are rather time-sensitive, and if not completed in a specific time, it results in immediate implications. While these tasks are not important to you, they are important to someone else and important to them in achieving their goal. Using Eisenhower's Urgent/Important Principle, you can structure your to-do list to prioritize things that are urgent and important first before working your way down to the tasks that are neither important nor urgent. When scheduling your time and constructing your to-do list, if you find tasks that are neither important nor urgent, you could easily mark these up as being time wasters and remove them from your schedule entirely. You can then work on prioritizing urgent and important tasks and trying to plan for the future to ensure that the next tasks don't become urgent but rather are completed before they become a pressed-for-time task.

## Step Six: Plan Ahead

There have been so many days where I have had so many things to do that I didn't even know where to begin. I would bounce between two or more tasks, some that were important and others that were urgent, and by the end of the day, I would have started five different tasks and not completed a single one. I am sure that I am not the only one who has experienced such days.

Nevertheless, the only way I was able to fix this was by planning.

Something that I have made a necessary and important part of my day is to make my to-do list and plan the following day down to a tee. It may seem overboard, but I even include my coffee breaks and my lunch breaks, and what I plan on eating during lunchtime. With a plan set in place, any uncertainty for the next day is almost entirely removed. I know what my priorities are for the next day, I know what I need to achieve, and I know what tasks have spilled into the next day from the previous day. If I didn't finish something today, I try to figure out why I allowed myself to let this task go by incomplete. Perhaps it wasn't urgent, but it was important. If it is important, it means it has to get completed the next day, and if it is urgent, it needs to be at the top of the to-do list.

Something else that always seems to disrupt our plans, our priorities, or our to-do lists are those unplanned circumstances that always seem to creep in. Whether it is a power outage, forgetting your keys at home, an accident on the road, or, even worse, a sick kid, there are days when a wrench gets thrown into our works and seems to take us almost entirely off track for what we were hoping to achieve. What I try to do is set aside an extra half an hour, which is a floating time slot, into my schedule each day. This means that, should anything unexpected arise, I could consider cutting down on my coffee break or my lunch break, and that time, coupled with the half an hour I have set aside, can be used to take care of any crisis that arises.

There are some days when my child is sick, my dog needs to be taken to the vet, or we face the loss of a loved one where half an hour is not going to help in those days. I often get asked what I do in those instances. The only thing you can do in those moments is to realize and acknowledge that you are human, and you allow yourself the time and the space to deal with what is going on around you. We can plan as much as we want to, but the reality is that we are never fully in control of every aspect of our lives. In those unavoidable, unplanned, and all-consuming moments, you need to give yourself the time to experience what you need to without the consequences of facing your own personal repercussions.

There is a famous saying that states that failing to plan is planning to fail. But why is that so? When you do not plan, you are immediately failing to manage your time. You are going about your day completely blind, and you have no expectations or preparations for the day. When you don't have a plan, you give yourself the illusion of falling behind, you feel like you are losing control, and because you have no plan, you have no way of comparing where you are with where you began. This all causes a downward spiral and can lead to burnout even faster.

With a simple plan in your hand, you may not conquer the world, but you can conquer your world.

## Step Seven: Give Every Project a Deadline

Deadlines. When you read that word, it may make your heart beat slightly faster. It is often associated with something big and scary, and it usually forms a trigger in our minds of something terrifying. This negativity forms in relation to the word "deadline" because we have fought hard to meet them, we have missed them, which has led to repercussions, or we have felt like failures when missing deadlines on collaborative projects. But deadlines play such an important role in getting our minds to focus and achieve something we are working on.

If you think about it, if something didn't have a deadline, we'd probably forget about it and never work on it, and it would never get done. A lot of people that I speak to tell me this about their passion projects. These projects are ones that they want to complete. They love doing it, but it is purely for them. So, instead, the things that they have to do usually take priority over the things that they want to do, and they never get around to doing what they want to do.

I have a friend who really enjoys pottery. She doesn't do it because she has to, but she rather does it because she wants to. She has all the equipment in the comfort of her home, so she never needs to go anywhere for pottery; she doesn't need to pay for classes, and she doesn't need to answer anyone about what she is doing. But this just means that she has no one to answer to. When I last spoke to her, she hadn't worked on any new pottery projects in the last three months, despite having all the resources available to her at her fingertips.

Having personal deadlines holds you accountable to yourself. If you know you need to complete something by a certain time, you know you can consciously work hard to achieve that goal. But it doesn't just help on a personal level. Deadlines form a great foundation for professional and academic collaborations.

In a professional setting, if you work with a group of people, each may have their own way of doing things and carrying out tasks. But having a deadline allows everyone to unite and work toward a common goal. For example, you may have someone who works at their own pace and sets aside time each day to work on a particular project. Then you may have someone who completes the entire project in the space of two days right before the deadline. No matter how each person works, by the time the deadline rolls around, each person will have completed what was exactly expected from them.

From an academic perspective, projects are all set according to milestones and deadlines. This is because certain requirements are expected to be met for the institution to keep track of progress and grades that a person may achieve. Without deadlines, teachers or lecturers, students, and the institution are completely unlinked and uncoordinated.

It is in our basic human nature to do better and work harder under some sort of pressure, and deadlines create this much-needed pressure that helps us work better. Personally, I work hard toward a deadline so that I can enjoy the rest that comes from the day after the deadline. That is the day when your stress levels drop, and you get to enjoy the peace and silence.

When setting deadlines, I have seen with myself and with many others around me that setting deadlines for every task, big or small, proves to be extremely beneficial. We know the importance of deadlines in the professional and workplace setting, but what about at home? What I tend to do is set deadlines for myself on a personal level. For example, I tell myself that we are having guests over for dinner at 6:00 p.m., which means that by 5:30 p.m., all the dishes that are currently in the sink need to be done and packed away. I also tell myself that bedtime for my kids is at 9:00 p.m., which means that at 8:00 p.m., bath time needs to be done. Through these deadlines, my family and I have created a structured and productive daily routine at home.

## Never Underestimate Time Management

We have all probably seen countless online courses promoting time management classes to teach people the valuable skills of managing the greatest commodity around. I, for one, used to quickly scroll past or ignore such ads because, ironically, I didn't have the time to dedicate to a time management course. But, in fact, when adhered to, applied to, and implemented correctly into our lifestyles, we may experience large amounts of success in managing our time.

Time management is underestimated, and the reason for that is that the results of any and all time management techniques are not immediate. As human beings, we want to see results immediately; we want to know right away if something is working, but time management takes time.

If I could share one piece of valuable advice to the working woman who is concerned that she may experience burnout, it would be to never underestimate the value of time management. Time management means scheduling everything. Scheduling everything is vital because it even allows you to schedule downtime and relaxation time.

# Chapter 6

# Mindfulness—Blocking Out Burnout Once and for All

We've already spoken about the feeling of driving home for an hour and getting home only to realize that you don't remember anything from the drive. We are all familiar with the feeling of being somewhat lost inside our own minds and getting lost in our thoughts or feeling like we're floating through reality, completely unaware of what's happening around us and to us. We feel shrouded by the cloud of our minds and almost weighed down by something that isn't even physical.

This feeling that many are familiar with is the feeling of not being entirely mindful or present at the moment.

But what is mindfulness? It may seem like a strange concept with our minds constantly working and being ever present with us, but being mindful is not an automatic response, believe it or not. Mindfulness is the human ability to be fully aware of what is occurring around us and within us; we are aware of what we are doing and why we are doing it, and we do it with a purpose, so we are not overly reactive and overwhelmed by the circumstances (Mindful Staff, 2020).

According to Professor Mark Williams, mindfulness means knowing what is going on inside and outside of ourselves each moment of every day.

Mindfulness has been closely associated with meditation, and a lot of the time, people confuse the two or expect them to be the same thing. However, this is not true. One can be a causality of the other, but they are most certainly not the same thing. People often use meditation as a tool to achieve mindfulness or mindfulness as a way to better their meditation practices.

While there are different approaches that work for different people, mindfulness has been highlighted as one of the best ways of minimizing burnout in addition to time management. The reason for this is that when you are mindful, you are conscious and aware of what is going on around you, you are alert, and you know the tasks you need to get through, rather than just guessing and assuming. When you are mindful, you know what you have to do and what you need to do.

Mindfulness, being closely related to meditation, has been found to hold a false sense of spirituality. It is a false thought that you have to follow new-age spiritual beliefs in order to take part in mindful practices, but this is a false notion that I hope to debunk to some extent for those who may be hesitant about employing mindfulness practices as a means of reducing the chances of becoming burnt out. Some people assume that you have to follow a specific belief system or religion to engage in mindfulness, but this is not true. Mindfulness, although considered a spiritual practice, can be part of some of the most basic or the most complex components of your life. When I talk about simple components, I mean that you can be mindful about going to the grocery store. In doing so, you will know and be conscious about what you are walking in to buy. If you have a list in hand, you may try to stick to that list as best you can, and you may be mindful of the budget you are hoping to stick to. But on an even smaller level, you will be mindful, aware, and alert of your surroundings; you will make sure that you don't push the grocery cart into others near you.

When you head out for a walk, you are mindful of your actions. You are present in the moment. It allows you to enjoy the company of those who may be with you on your walk, and it introduces an element of safety into this type of interaction. You are aware of who is around you, if there is anything to be suspicious of, and if your mind can maintain its calm. You may find yourself acutely aware of staying far from the curb because you have your child with you.

Being mindful and aware in the professional setting will ensure things get accomplished on a certain day. It will be making sure that you know what tasks you have to address and what projects you need to complete and having a plan, either written or mental, on how you plan to approach and complete these tasks. Mindfulness is especially beneficial when you are collaborating and working with others in that you are aware of their time. This makes you work harder and push harder at certain tasks.

For me to have a better understanding of mindfulness, I like to think of it as taking out your earphones when there are people talking to you, and you need to focus on a task. The loud music in your ears may take your focus away from what you're doing, people can't talk to you, and you feel overwhelmed by everything happening. Taking out your earphones makes you feel like you are suddenly awake and able to fully immerse yourself in what you are doing.

Now, while mindfulness may help you physically achieve tasks and help you stay alert and aware of your surroundings, and while it does make you purposeful in your actions and how you interact and relate with others, you may be wondering how it helps with your overall health and well-being on an internal level.

How does mindfulness help you keep your mind healthy? When you are mindful of everything happening around you and when you remove yourself from your thoughts, you may find it easier to stop stressing and to stop your strong and overpowering feelings of anxiety. When you are mindful, you are able to notice the changes that are occurring inside your body as a first response. Through mindfulness, you are able to pay attention to everything happening within your body. When you have a mindful approach to yourself, you become acutely aware of your stress cycles and where you are in your stress cycles, and you are able to stop it from escalating beyond your control—all of these because you are now more in tune with, aware of, and mindful of your body.

To some, mindfulness may seem like a weird concept, especially for those who have type A personalities and who are often more aggressive and hard on themselves. But everyone can practice and employ mindful tactics to reduce stress. Using mindfulness can allow you to be more compassionate with yourself, and treating yourself with this compassion and understanding limits the amount of stress you allow into your space. But there are many ways that mindfulness can reduce stress (Mindful Staff, 2021):

You become more aware of and more attuned to your thoughts. Do you know those negative thoughts that you keep hearing inside your head? That little voice is you. You are telling yourself all the negative things that send you into a flat spin, and that causes you a lot of stress. When you become more aware of your thoughts, you give yourself the space to step back and look at your thoughts with some sense of awareness. You can rationalize what you are thinking, and you can ask yourself if such thoughts are warranted. When you remove yourself ever so slightly from your thoughts, you allow yourself not to take them so literally, and you prevent your stress response from even appearing in the first place. Do you know that thought that pops into your head that if you don't meet a deadline, you are going to lose your job? That thought is stopped in its tracks by asking your superiors for an extension if needed.

You give yourself the space to pause before impulsively reacting to a situation. There are many things that trigger off our stress response, and in particular, there are situations that evoke extreme and sometimes irrational responses. When you employ a mindful approach and mindful strategies, you give yourself the space to stop, assess, and think about the situation before reacting to it. Let me give you an example: If you are in a shopping center parking lot and someone opens their door into your car, your immediate response may be to lash out, yell, and perhaps negatively and impulsively use behavior that is extremely unlike you. However, when you are mindful, you will pause and take a deep breath, and you may save yourself a really horrible story to tell. When you act impulsively, you create the possibility of giving really mean and nasty responses to people. In my own personal pursuit of mindfulness, I have found putting myself in the shoes of the person who would be on the receiving end of my impulsivity. I ask myself what they might be going through; perhaps they have a sick family member and are rushing to the drugstore. Maybe they have recently lost a loved one. Maybe they are so severely under stress that they are nearing burnout. What if my actions are what sets them off? Mindfulness has really helped me think of the other person. When you are mindful, you are also available to better understand the emotions of others. Your sense of empathy is increased, and your overall emotional intelligence is higher.

You activate the "being" mode and deactivate the "doing" mode of your mind. You have two modes of operation as a human. The being mode is associated with being calm and relaxed, and the doing mode is executing an action and even activating your stress response. When you flow through the motion of things, and you are not mindful of what you are doing, you just do. You are not aware, and you are not focused. However, when you are "being," you are actively involved in every aspect of the task at hand. But the being mode also allows you to remember that you are human and that you are allowed to take breaks. It makes sure you understand that the resting version of you is the best thing for the tasks you will take on in the future.

You become more aware of the needs and the demands of your body. The one thing that I have been talking about throughout this entire book is making sure that you are aware of your body so that you can stop stress and burnout before it even happens. That is exactly what mindfulness does. It allows you to listen to your body better. When you are aware of your body and its internal and physical feelings, you experience pain, emotions, and feelings of anxiety a lot sooner so that you can begin acting on it faster and begin taking action to stop any damage to your body. You can stop the stress before it spirals out of control.

You will find yourself being more compassionate to yourself and to others. Being a more compassionate version of yourself allows you to suppress your own stress response. We tell ourselves that, as parents, we need to take a more gentle approach in dealing with our kids. Yelling at them is in no way an appropriate response to certain types of unwanted behavior. Saying mean things is not appropriate at all. So why do we think it's okay to do this to ourselves? Compassion toward ourselves makes stress a lot less because we portray a sense of understanding toward the emotions, and we are active in finding solutions for any problem rather than feeling guilty and overwhelmed.

Mindfulness calms down the amygdala. Mindfulness helps us activate a physiological response in our brain by reducing the activity that takes place in the amygdala. The amygdala is also the area of the brain that triggers our stress response. If this activity is reduced, your all-around stress response will be reduced.

Mindfulness enhances focus. When you are mindful, you can focus better, and when you can focus better, you are able to work better and you are able to be more efficient and more effective in carrying out the task at hand. There is an obvious and direct link between focusing better and reducing stress. Greater focus equals less stress, which makes the pursuit of mindfulness much more appealing to the person struggling to fight the burnout that they may experience.

You can rationalize your stress and use it as a source of motivation. We have already mentioned that some sort of pressure pushes us to work harder. When you are mindful, you reassess your stress, and you face it in a more rational way. When you take on a mindful approach, you can turn your stress around from holding negative connotations, and you can use it as a positive driving force and motivation.

## Being Mindful

Now that we have seen the benefits of mindfulness, how can you achieve mindfulness, and what are the best mindfulness practices for you to employ? I am glad you asked. As we have mentioned before, meditation is a great way to gain mindfulness. Through meditation, you expand your mind as if you are sailing on the waters of a calm ocean. You get to experience and fully embrace the stillness that comes with mindfulness which creates increased peace and calmness in your mind. But there are other ways of achieving mindfulness. One of the ways which I have found to be the most common in achieving mindfulness is through breathing. Breathing exercises that are focused and intentional make your mind calmer. The next thing you can do to achieve mindfulness is to reconnect with nature. Taking walks outside will not only help with those breathing exercises by filling your lungs with fresh air, but it will also allow you to reconnect with yourself. You will find yourself fully enjoying a seemingly basic task. You take joy in the steps, and you enjoy a task that would otherwise seem like too much effort.

Another important aspect of achieving mindfulness is allowing yourself to take breaks throughout your day and avoid multitasking. If you are overloaded, your mind doesn't have the chance to be fully present in the moment. Instead, it is trying to figure out what task to focus on. Everything takes priority which means you're juggling many things, and nothing gets the attention it actually deserves. When you take breaks, you give yourself the mental offload that it needs by stepping away from the things that may be draining your energy. And when you focus on one thing at a time, you can complete the task from start to end and tick a completed item off your to-do list.

Mindfulness comes from taking a moment and living completely in the moment. Living in the moment is fine and well, so long as you are doing it mindfully. Yes, it may sound strange to hear that you are not living consciously, but while the focus and emphasis have been placed on your surroundings and while you're living in the moment, take time to introspect and be happy with yourself. You need to be mindful of who you are at the moment, and during that moment, there is absolutely no change you can make to the person you currently are. You need to appreciate yourself for where you are, how you are doing, and how far you have come, and appreciate the fact that you are still motivated to carry on. You need to acknowledge that even though you may be stressed these days, you are taking steps to avoid burnout from happening. Finding yourself in your own mind and accepting yourself is the greatest step toward mindfulness, and mindfulness is a great step toward avoiding burnout.

Steps toward mindfulness also aid you in becoming a calmer and more refreshed version of yourself. Remember that a journey toward mindfulness is a journey toward complete avoidance of burnout. This is not a one-time task. It is something that you consistently work toward. The world will never stop throwing stress at us, so we should never stop working toward achieving and maintaining mindfulness.

Staying abreast of technology can also help on the journey toward mindfulness. There have been many mindfulness applications that have been developed and launched, but whether or not they work, figuring out which one is best depends on the person who is planning to use the app. As with our limits, how fast we get burnt out, and our mindfulness journeys, the use of apps, or even technology as a whole, is a very individualistic thing. For those who find themselves extremely disciplined and who work well not being accountable to other people, a mobile application may work great for them. Those who need help and encouragement from others may not find themselves benefiting from an app but rather from a face-to-face and guided meditation session.

Perhaps we have been asking the wrong questions regarding mindfulness and meditation apps. The questions should not be whether they work or not but should rather be why they work for some people and not for other people. However, whatever means a person uses; we could all benefit from being a little more mindful.

# Chapter 7

# Enjoy Your Job Again

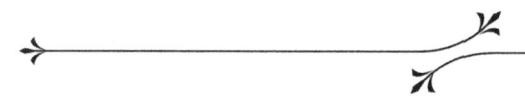

A good old saying states, "If you enjoy your job, you will never work a day in your life." But sometimes, the feelings of stress and overwhelm can cause us to experience feelings of resentment toward our jobs. If we are not currently feeling it, we may have felt it in the past—the feeling of waking up and absolutely despising our job. Some people hate what they do, and whether they are just in it for the money or not, they really don't want to be working in that job. They hate their job so much that waking up in the morning is the hardest thing they have to do. With hatred being such a strong word and such a powerful feeling, staying in a job that you hate can quickly lead you to become burnt out, purely because the emotional stress and pressure of the job are too much for you. People don't just hate their jobs because they think they aren't getting paid enough. People hate their jobs because of poor leadership; they hate the task or the monotony of what they are doing each day; they may hate the people that they work with, or they may hate the environment in which they work. I know using the word hate is really strong, but when you are familiar with the feeling of dissatisfaction with your job, "hate" seems like the only way to describe it.

Nigel Marsh, the author of *Fat, Forty, and Fired*, states that being in a job that you hate can cause more mental instabilities than you may experience being unemployed. Wow! Can you imagine that? Being unemployed in any economic climate is extremely stressful. We have families to take care of, so the greatest concern that arises is finances, and we are faced with extreme pressure overall.

Being unemployed is the complete opposite of what this book is about. In this book, I am aiming to help those women who are working so hard that they seem like they just might snap. Being unemployed is about having the drive to work and the willingness to work; it is looking at someone who may be experiencing burnout and thinking that you'd rather have that than be unemployed. These two extreme ends are on the same scale, and each is concerning in its own right.

Being happy in your job is so important, but again, having someone telling you not to stress in an extremely stressful situation and telling you to be happy with your job seems like something you have no control over. Being happy with your job is not something that you can directly control. You can also really enjoy and love what you do but still, experience burnout. The thing about being happy with and loving your job is that you may not identify that you are burnt out because the love for your job is so strong. This is both a good and a bad thing.

Happiness is an internal emotion, but it greatly influences our actions. If you are feeling unhappy with your job, it is important to know why so that you can take steps to change this. Life is too short to stay in a job that you are unhappy with. If your compensation is not enough, then maybe you need to speak to your superiors about possible growth and development within the company. If you are unhappy with the daily tasks that you are required to complete, perhaps changing departments may be the best solution for you. If you are not happy with the environment that you are in, and you feel as though the mental toll is too high to stay in this job, maybe leave and step away from this position, even if you don't have something in the pipeline just as yet, may be the best option.

If you feel unhappy with your job and you feel lost or stuck, do not fret. I have some key tips that you can use which may make you fall in love with your job again—and that is something that may help you avoid burnout. But before I start with these tips, there are a few things you need to know. I've said it previously, and I will say it again: People get burnt out even if they are doing a job that they love and that they enjoy. In fact, identifying burnout when you are doing your favorite job may be harder than if you are doing a job you know you don't like. The next thing I need you to know is that if you can't see yourself falling in love with your job or you don't want to fall in love with your job, do not be afraid to begin searching for something new. Do not be afraid of walking away.

Now, let us delve into the little steps you can take toward enjoying your job again.

Find something you like. Yes, when you get home after a long day at work, you have a long list of things to complain about, which is a list of all the things you hate. But maybe you could switch and change the narrative. Find one thing about your job that you don't hate, and use that to change how you feel about your position. Even if it is your colleagues that make everything a little more bearable, think of them in the difficult moments. When you are carrying out a task that stresses you out a lot, take a walk to your colleagues' desks, and ask them how their day is going. Maybe you really enjoy one aspect of your job and just hate another. Perhaps you love doing presentations, but you hate the preparation that goes into getting ready for a presentation. Use the end product of the final presentation as your motivating factor to enjoy the task you are not looking forward to. Finding goodness and positivity in anything can ease the weight on your shoulders.

1. Define the purpose and the goal of your job. Something that is really important to remember is that your job is not the goal. Your job is a means to achieving a goal. We are not living to work, and we shouldn't live our lives focused on what we hope to achieve from a job. Instead, our jobs are a secondary aspect of our lives that are meant to fund the things we enjoy doing. So set a new motivating factor behind your job. Perhaps you want to go on holiday, or you want to build something new in your home. Changing your goal and changing something you are working toward can be enough to motivate you once more.
2. Create a social element at work. We are social beings, after all. Have lunch with a colleague, go out for a coffee with someone, and spend some time with the people at work rather than just the work. Often, we don't realize that the people at work may look up to us, we may be the motivation behind them working hard, or they may appreciate the small things you do that make their job easier. The only way that you may be able to find out or explore

such possibilities is by actually connecting and communicating with your colleagues.

3. Determine what you hate about your job. Figuring out exactly what it is about the work that makes you not want to wake up in the morning is the only way to remedy the feeling itself. But remember that lines can easily be blurred. If you don't like doing certain tasks of your job, that negativity may bleed into other aspects, and you may find yourself thinking that you don't enjoy the people or the management in your company. That is why it is first and foremost important to figure out what you don't like about your job.

4. Learn a new skill. Monotony is enough to make you feel stagnant and stuck. It is enough to make you feel like you really don't want to go to work. Maybe try learning something new. It can be directly related to what you do, or it can be a new hobby. Learning something new will feel like a breath of fresh air.

5. Ask, and you shall receive. "Do you know what is going on with Nelly?" "Do you know why Ollie seems a bit more riled up today compared to usual?" No, you don't, because they haven't told you. The same goes for you. Your manager, superior, or colleagues may not know that you are on the verge of burnout; they may not know that you hate your job, and they may not know that you are facing financial difficulties and may need a wage increase. It is

important to be open and vocal about what you are feeling about your job. They may be able to assist you in achieving happiness again with your job.
6. No more negativity. It is easy to get caught up in office gossip or get pulled into conversations that are made up of complaining about managers and other colleagues, but for your own mental health, you need to stay away from such negativity and surround yourself with positivity. If you hear such conversations arising around the water cooler, do yourself a favor and step away. Take the time to nurture yourself and your growth because, at the end of the day, the negative talks are in no way going to add to your life.
7. Take breaks as and when you need them. Burnout is not some figment of your imagination, it is not something that has been created by lazy people, and it is difficult to overcome. You need to do whatever it takes to protect yourself and your mental health from burnout and the devastating effects it leaves in its wake. In modern workplaces, a lot of companies and people in management positions are acknowledging the effects of mental health illnesses and burnout, and some companies are even including mental health days which allow employees to take a break for their own mental health. Go on a road trip over the weekend, plan a getaway, and take your vacation days. While it may not be feasible to go on an annual vacation abroad

every year, try to take a little break here and there to benefit your mind and soul.
8. Many companies offer a wide variety of benefits—take them. If your place of employment offers mental health days, if they offer gym memberships, or if they give you exclusive access to a specific coffee shop just by working there, take advantage of it! People don't take advantage of some benefits because they think they may be saving the company some money, but if a company is offering you some sort of benefit and perk, chances are they have the capacity and feasibility to do so. Take advantage of your benefits. If your company pays for you to see a therapist as and when you need it, that is something you should use with pleasure.
9. Start a side project. This side project could either be a side hustle or a hobby. If it is a side hustle, you may start it as a ramp-up project until it gains enough traction to sustain you, and you can leave your day job. Sometimes our day job is just what we need to fund our dream job. If it is a hobby, it may just be what you need to get in touch with yourself again, to start your mindfulness journey, or to give yourself the mental break that you need after pushing yourself to your own mental limits almost on a daily basis. A side project can be great for you on every level if you are open to the idea.
10. And lastly, if nothing from the list works, you may need to take the leap into looking for another job

and looking for another place of work. Yes, job hunting is stressful, but if none of the above steps seems like it will work for you if you do truly hate your job, and if it just weighs down way too heavy on you, perhaps you need to ask yourself if the stress of finding a new job or even being unemployed for a short period of time is greater than or less than the stress you are currently undergoing. Maybe taking this big jump into the unknown and this big leap of faith is exactly what you need to venture away from burnout and toward maintaining your mental health.

By reading this book, I am sure you can see how passionate I am about women experiencing burnout. Avoiding burnout is a primary concern of mine, and it should be for everyone. If avoiding burnout means taking a big risk to save your mental health, I think it is worth it. There are always things to consider and things to note. I am not advising you to make an irrational decision to hand in your resignation tomorrow, but perhaps this is the push you need to start having conversations with your partner and start looking at your current financial situation in considering whether or not you and your family may be in a safe position for you to walk away from a job until you find something new. Sometimes we look for signs or an answer to these questions. Maybe this is your sign.

# How to Ease Your Workload

Ultimately, our stress stems from us carrying more than our shoulders can withstand. Yes, we can pile more and more onto the load, and it will get heavier and heavier, but at some point, either our back, knees, or shoulders are bound to give up under the load. But if you ask someone to help, maybe they can take one or two things off your shoulders and help you carry the load.

There are many times when we feel like asking for help may make us seem weak or vulnerable, but asking for help can actually be seen as something brave that takes courage to do, and it shows that you are confident enough in your abilities to know your limits and boundaries. Asking for help can be beneficial not only in easing the load on your shoulders but also in building and creating connections with others. When you ask someone for help, you show them that you trust them and their capabilities in assisting you with something that is extremely important to you. This is a great way of forming a connection with a family member or a colleague at work.

Just like apologizing, asking for help is really difficult for some people. The reason for this stems from multiple possible reasons. The first is that they may have been taught that asking for help is a bad thing. A lot of the time, people think that if you ask for help, your capabilities will be questioned. People think that if you ask for help, you are seen as weak. In the workplace, some people may avoid asking for help because they fear their superiors may think they are incapable of carrying out certain tasks. But this is definitely not the case.

Another reason why people may not want to ask for help is that they are uncomfortable or because they are shy. We have all been to a presentation or a class, and we have all heard someone say, "Please feel free to ask anything. There are no stupid questions." But just because the lecturer or speaker has said this does not mean that the shy person at the back of the room is suddenly going to gain the confidence to ask a question. In their mind, the question may still be stupid. They may be an introvert, or they may be terrified to speak in front of others. Asking for help in these instances is just all-around hard for the person.

The last reason why some people may not ask for help is that their ego won't allow them to. Some people think way too highly of themselves, and they would never want to risk asking for help if it would make others think they are not the absolute best. These are the people who often do themselves a disservice, and they are the ones who look down on others who may ask for help.

But what would be the solution for people in either of these circumstances? Well, a quick rephrasing of words can make even the most haughty person a bit more comfortable with a task they may be facing. For example, if someone is not comfortable asking for help, they may approach the whole situation in a different way. They may find themselves approaching others and asking for input and ideas on a project they are working on. Through this collaborative process, they are able to achieve input from different points of view; they are able to consider aspects that may have never previously crossed their mind; they are able to indirectly ease their mental load. They are able to do all of this without explicitly asking for help.

On the basis of being a fully functioning and successful human being, it is important to realize that asking for help is important no matter who you are, what you can do, and even what you can't do. Having a great title doesn't mean you can't ask for help, and it also doesn't mean that no one will help you if you ask.

As a working mother, I found it difficult to ask for help, even when I just couldn't do things for myself. I didn't avoid asking for help because of fear or because of my ego but rather because I felt that certain things were my responsibility and needed to be done by me. For example, I needed to revise patient paperwork because it gets updated every six months, any changes in health history need to be documented; and as one of the providers treating the patient, it was part of my job to make sure all documentation was scanned, and that it was in the right patient's file. Then, when I would get home after work, I would feel that it was my job to cook dinner and do the dishes. Either this was because I always did it or because I felt this was the role I had to assume. Dinner and dishes were on me. Next, I would be the one to bathe, dress, and put my kids to bed. Don't get me wrong; this is one thing I really love doing, but there were many times that I was filling the bathtub while checking on the pots, and the food would end up burnt. But I felt like it was my duty to bathe the kids because they were my responsibility. After all, I couldn't place the responsibility of my kids onto someone else. But this is where my thoughts needed to be adjusted.

At work, yes, I have responsibilities that can't be transferred to somebody else, things like educating the patient, guiding them on where to go when they are referred out, or what is next after they are seen by the specialist. But laying out the workspace and all the tools I need to use, despite wanting it set out in a specific way, could be done by someone else. I had to ask for help, and while some x-rays were taken or some stocking was done, I could finish any paperwork, any scanning, or information that needed to be sent to the patient's insurance or anything that needed to be done for my previous patient. Next, I needed to ask for help with cooking and with my kids. I had to split the duty and realized that I was not a superwoman. While I handled dinner, my partner would sort out the kids' night routine, or we would swap.

Admitting to myself and to others that it was fine to need help and to ask for help was a complete game changer.

# Conclusion

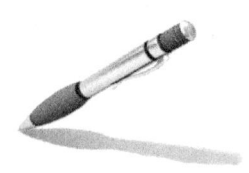

Now that you have reached the end of this book, you may have the immediate urge to start doing what you have learned here. You may even already be reaching for a pen and paper to start making your to-do list. But wait! You need to know that anything worth doing and worth achieving takes time. Avoiding burnout is not something you are going to start and finish right now. Some days will be harder, and some days will be easier. But the key is to keep on working at maintaining your own personal balance. In addition, comparing yourself to anyone else in this world is a disservice to you and to the other person. There is no other you in this world but you. So just because your colleague does even more than you and they are not burnt out does not mean you need to start a race that was never meant to be run.

Now that you have an understanding of stress and burnout and now that it is a fully formulated thought in your mind, you can better understand its relation to you and to your life. You know when you need to keep an eye on your body to look out for symptoms of stress because you are expecting a deadline or you are attending a high-profile event. You know when and how to monitor yourself for symptoms of stress, and you now have the ability to intercept these symptoms before they grab hold of you entirely in an all-consuming death grip.

But even if you do find yourself sinking, you will now know how to use mindful practices, time management, and other mechanisms to self-regulate and stop your stress cycle dead in its tracks.

# Accepting Yourself

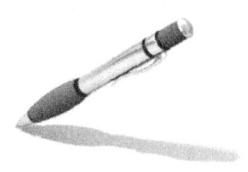

If there was only one thing that I would like you to take away from this, it would be learning from the experiences that have led to burnout, in yourself or in others, and realizing that even the best and greatest of people in the world have experienced burnout. You are not a failure when you are exhausted. As a mother or as a professional, I always felt like a failure in either one or the other way. Either I was giving too much attention to my job, or I was focusing too much on my kids and neglecting my work. I felt like a failure, and I felt constantly worn out and worn thin. That is until I realized that my priorities needed adjusting.

I am the person who would do anything for her family and who would do anything for her patients. That is my makeup as a human being and my personality, and that is fine. There are some days when I may not be able to meet anyone else's needs but my own, and there are days when the only needs I may be able to meet are my partner's and my kid's. And the guilt from the built-up stress will tell me that it makes me a bad professional.

But I took control of that little voice in my mind, and I responded with, "I am not a bad professional. I am a great human being."

We need to learn self-love, self-care, and self-appreciation. Taking time out for yourself, eating a meal alone or catching up with your friends, and taking time away from the many roles that you are already filling as a professional and a mother, does not make you bad at anything. It is a fundamental part of maintaining your sanity and avoiding burnout. You can take a night off from being a superwoman because even superheroes need to gather themselves and take a break from all the difficulties that life brings.

But also, make no mistake in assuming that burnout has its pick between men and women. Undoubtedly, there seems to be greater societal pressure on women than on men. If you are a working mother, you are expected to return home after your "first shift" and begin your "second shift," which entails taking care of your family and your home. In a study conducted in 2019, it was found that women were at a 39% greater risk of experiencing burnout than their male counterparts (Malesic, 2022).

But men do experience burnout in a different way. The type of societal pressure that weighs heavy on the shoulder of a man is far different from that of a woman. They are expected to not show a single smidgen of weakness, which often leads to them feeling overstressed and, yes, burnt out. They are not exempt from experiencing burnout but, instead, do experience it in ways far different than women do. And while this book focuses on professional women who may be experiencing burnout, it will not ignore that men and stay-at-home moms are not immune to burnout.

Maybe the realization that may come with you reading this book is not just the great ways of avoiding burnout, but rather, it allows you to take a gentler approach to those around you. Maybe after reading this book, you will treat everyone with a gentler approach and a more mindful approach, and when they are the ones to ask you for help, you can look at them with a knowing smile and gladly offer them the assistance they need. As a parent, maybe this is what helps you raise a gentler child, someone who understands the feelings of those around them. And if that, dear reader, is all you take away from this book and you save yourself or someone else from experiencing the world-shattering effects of burnout, then I have successfully done what I have intended to do.

# References

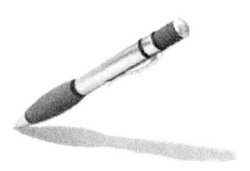

Cassoobhoy, A. (2020, December 13). What is cortisol? WebMD. https://www.webmd.com/a-to-z-guides/what-is-cortisol

CFI Team. (2022, May 7). SMART Goal - Definition, guide, and importance of goal setting. Corporate Finance Institute. https://corporatefinanceinstitute.com/resources/knowledge/other/smart-goal/

Dike, C. (2017, June 29). Stress vs. burnout–What's the difference. Doctor On Demand. https://blog.doctorondemand.com/stress-vs-burnout-whats-the-difference-429547f5d82a

Dreamcloud Editorial Team. (2019, July 15). 10 Healthy coping mechanisms to manage stress. DreamCloud. https://www.dreamcloudsleep.com/posts/healthy-coping-mechanisms/

Freudenberger, H. J. (1975). The staff burn-out syndrome in alternative institutions. Psychotherapy:

Theory, Research & Practice, 12(1), 73–82. https://doi.org/10.1037/h0086411

GoodTherapy. (2018, September 26). Coping mechanisms. https://www.goodtherapy.org/blog/psychpedia/coping-mechanisms

Håkansson, M. (2013, March 15). Signs you're disconnected from your body + what to do about it. MindBodyGreen. https://www.mindbodygreen.com/0-8119/signs-youre-disconnected-from-your-body-what-to-do-about-it.html

Hanh, T. N. (n.d.). Five steps to mindfulness. https://uhs.berkeley.edu/sites/default/files/article_-_five_steps_to_mindfulness.pdf

Johns Hopkins Medicine. (2021, April 27). Bruxism. https://www.hopkinsmedicine.org/health/conditions-and-diseases/bruxism#:~:text=Mouthguard

Jones, K. P. (2017). What exactly are syndromes? Utah.edu. https://healthcare.utah.edu/the-scope/shows.php?shows=0_398izmir

Lawson, K. (n.d.). Why it's important to master stress. Taking Charge of Your Health & Wellbeing.

https://www.takingcharge.csh.umn.edu/why-its-important-master-stress

Malesic, J. (2022, January 4). Opinion | How burnout affects men. The New York Times. https://www.nytimes.com/2022/01/04/opinion/burnout-men-signs.html

Marks, J. (2018, May 7). The stress response cycle. PsychCentral. https://psychcentral.com/blog/the-stress-reaction-cycle#1

Mayo Clinic Staff. (2021, June 5). Job burnout: How to spot it and take action. Mayo Clinic. https://www.mayoclinic.org/healthy-lifestyle/adult-health/in-depth/burnout/art-20046642

MedlinePlus. (2020, October 8). Stress and your health. https://medlineplus.gov/ency/article/003211.htm#:~:text=Stress%20is%20a%20feeling%20of

Mental Health Foundation. (2021, September 17). Stress. https://www.mentalhealth.org.uk/a-to-z/s/stress#:~:text=It%20is%20often%20triggered%20when

Mind Tools Content Team. (n.d.). Eisenhower's urgent/important principle: Using time effectively, not just efficiently. Mind Tools.

https://www.mindtools.com/pages/article/newHTE_91.htm#:~:text=The%20urgent%20are%20not%20important

Mind Tools Content Team. To-do lists: The key to efficiency. (n.d.a.). Mind Tools. https://www.mindtools.com/pages/article/newHTE_05.htm

Mindful Staff. (2020, July 8). What is mindfulness? Mindful. https://www.mindful.org/what-is-mindfulness/

Mindful Staff. (2021a, January 21). How to manage stress with mindfulness and meditation. Mindful. https://www.mindful.org/how-to-manage-stress-with-mindfulness-and-meditation/#:~:text=This%20compassionate%20mind%20soothes%20you

Moss, J. (2019, December 11). Burnout is about your workplace, not your people. Harvard Business Review. https://hbr.org/2019/12/burnout-is-about-your-workplace-not-your-people

NHS. Breathing exercises for stress. (2021, February 2). https://www.nhs.uk/mental-health/self-help/guides-tools-and-activities/breathing-exercises-for-stress/

Samartano, M. (2018, May 7). The Stress Reaction Cycle. Psych Central. https://psychcentral.com/blog/the-stress-reaction-cycle#1

Scott, E. (2020, March 12). Relaxation response for reversing stress. Verywell Mind. https://www.verywellmind.com/what-is-the-relaxation-response-3145145

Scott, E. (2020a, October 21). Traits and attitudes that increase burnout risk. Verywell Mind. https://www.verywellmind.com/mental-burnout-personality-traits-3144514

Stress cycles: What they are and how to break them. (2020, December 17). Embrace Sexual Wellness. https://www.embracesexualwellness.com/esw-blog/stresscycles

Stressors. (n.d.). Centre for Studies on Human Stress. https://humanstress.ca/stress/what-is-stress/stressors/

The difference between a career and a job and why it's important. (n.d.). College of West Anglia. https://cwa.ac.uk/about/alumni/alumni-news/the-difference-between-a-career-and-a-job-and-why-its-important#:~:text=The%20main%20difference%20between%20a

Understanding the stress response. (2020, July 6). Harvard Health Publishing. https://www.health.harvard.edu/staying-healthy/understanding-the-stress-response

World Health Organization. (2019, May 28). Burn-out an "occupational phenomenon": International Classification of Diseases. https://www.who.int/news/item/28-05-2019-burn-out-an-occupational-phenomenon-international-classification-of-diseases#:~:text=%E2%80%9CBurn%2Dout%20is%20a%20syndrome

Printed in Great Britain
by Amazon